how to get
wheelyfit

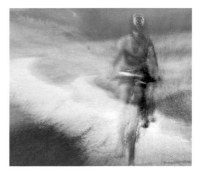

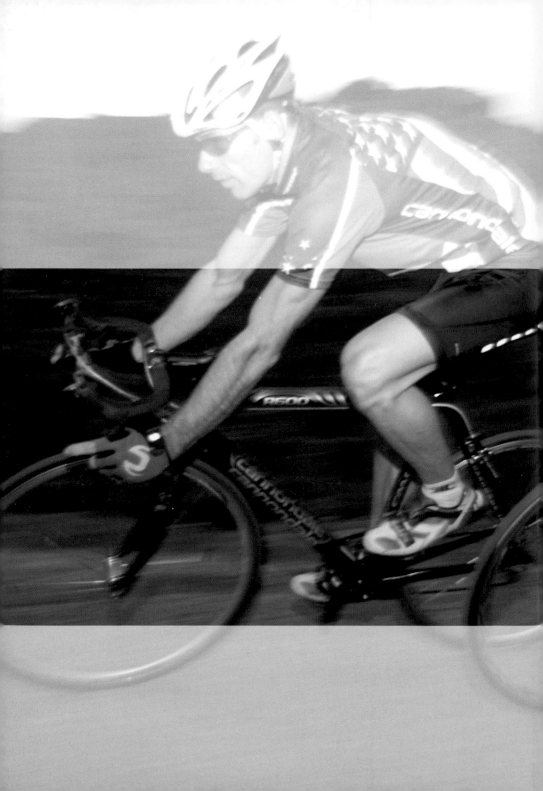

how to get
wheely fit

OLIVER ROBERTS

A CONNECTIONS • AXIS EDITION

A Connections • Axis Edition

This edition first published in Great
Britain by
Connections Book Publishing Limited
St Chad's House
148 King's Cross Road
London WC1X 9DH
and Axis Publishing Limited
8c Accommodation Road
London NW11 8ED
www.axispublishing.co.uk

Conceived and created by
Axis Publishing Limited

Creative Director: Siân Keogh
Designer: Axis Design Editions
Managing Editor: Brian Burns
Editor: Conor Kilgallon
Production Manager: Sue Bayliss
Production Controller: Juliet Brown
Photographer: Simon Punter

Text and images copyright
© Axis Publishing Limited 2003

Note
The opinions and advice expressed in
this book are intended as a guide only.
The publishers and author accept no
responsibility for any injury or loss
sustained as a result of using this book.

British Library Cataloguing-in-Publication
data available on request.

ISBN 1–85906–111–7

9 8 7 6 5 4 3 2 1

contents

how to get **wheely**fit

introduction

Imagine moving effortlessly along a quiet country lane. Woods, fields, and occasional houses slide past as the air rushes through your hair. You're

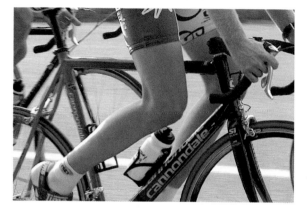

pedaling, but despite the speed, there's no real sense of effort. Your friends are beside you, chatting, and you smile to yourself, happy to be roaming the country on two wheels.

These feelings make cycling a sport of passion, a passion that appears in different guises. It appears as the screaming fans lining the route of the Tour de France as the whirring, rainbow spectacle of the professional teams race past. It is the willingness to pour body and soul into an effort to power your way up a climb or sprint the last miles of a time trial. It is the

the five types of cycling

touring

This is cycling at its most relaxed. Touring groups are usually unconcerned about pace, duration, or competition. They seek only the enjoyment of sunny days spent spinning through open country with a few friends.

1

road racing

The Tour de France, mountain climbs, sprints, the peleton... road-racing is often seen as something only exceptional athletes do. In fact, there are amateur races throughout the country organized in categories according to ability and experience, though you almost always need to be a club member and licensed to take part (see p. 11).

2

time trials

An off-shoot of the road-racing scene, time trials involve racing alone against the clock. Tough and fast, it's often called "the race of truth" because it's all up to individual strength.

3

irrepressible grin that spreads across your face as you fly effortlessly down a hill with your friends on a sunny morning. It is treating yourself to a really cool pair of shades.

But despite this passion, cycling is still a sport for everyone. It is also a great way to get fit, without the need for a gym, a trainer, or any organized teaching—all you really need is a bike and this book.

on the road

Cycling is a wonderfully simple activity—you get on your bike, push the pedals, and away you go. As a sport, it divides into a number of different areas (the main ones are outlined in the panel), but they all have the same root and it's easy to cross over between disciplines (indeed many riders do so, for the challenge and enjoyment of the different types of cycling).

This book deals mostly with road cycling because it is, in my opinion, the simplest and most popular type of cycling. This may sound strange given the popularity of mountain bikes, but many of those "off-road" bikes never see anything but tarmac. Be realistic— if you're going to do most of your riding on the road, buy a road bike. It will be faster, smoother, and a good deal less effort to pedal.

mountain biking

Off-road cycling at its most extreme. If you like mud, hurtling down woodland trails, and jumping obstacles, this is the one for you.

4

track

Speed is king on the track. Racing here is fast, furious, and extremely tactical. The bikes don't even have brakes!

5

in the saddle

Whether you want to find a calmer, more fun way to get to the office, shed a few pounds while socializing, or forge yourself into the next Lance Armstrong, cycling has something for you.

how to use this book

In the following chapters, you'll discover the secrets that will take you from total beginner to a fit, race-experienced cyclist.

Chapter 1 takes you through the tricky question of buying and fitting a bike. It dresses you in all the right clothing, as well as suggesting a few extra accessories you'll probably need. After that, it reveals the truth about food (what you should be eating and drinking for health and performance on

why cycle?

fitness
Regular activity makes your muscles, heart, and lungs stronger and work more efficiently. This makes daily chores easier, and you'll feel fitter and more energetic overall.

transport
Distances shrink, and places that you'd never try to walk to become ever more accessible. It's also clean and quiet, and you don't have to spend any money on gas or train tickets.

health
As little as 30 minutes of cycling three or four times a week will boost your general health, helping to prevent conditions such as heart disease and cancer.

relaxation
Exercise releases chemicals in our brains that calm us down and induce feelings of happiness.

self-confidence
Cycling is tremendously empowering. The sense of achievement you get from setting and reaching your goals, as well as the feelings of freedom and independence it engenders, are all great confidence boosters.

enjoyment
The world seems different on the back of a bicycle. Sights and sounds normally missed from inside a car leap out and take your breath away.

and off the bike), how to stay injury free, and how to keep yourself motivated (not that you'll need it once you're on your way!). Dip in and out of this chapter as you want.

Chapter 2 takes you into the world of training. After an overview of what training is and how it works, you'll find sections on developing specific skills. So whether you're trying to make it up that long climb a little quicker, or you want to know what to do when you go out on your first group ride, it's all here.

training schedules

The second half of chapter 2 takes you into training schedules, split into six levels (see opposite). If you've never ridden before, you can start at level one, and work your way up as far as you want. If you're a little more experienced to start with, you can jump in at the refresher course in level three.

Alternatively, pick up one of the goal-specific training programs, that cover everything from training to ride non stop for 100 miles (160 km), to breaking the hour-mark for a 25-mile (40-km) time trial. Levels three to six also have a basic training week that is designed to be repeated if you don't want to focus on competing.

schedules and levels

1 starter level 1

For total novices. From no riding or racing experience at all to riding for an hour, in four weeks.

2 starter level 2

For new riders ready for the next challenge. Trains you to ride comfortably for one hour non-stop, three or four times a week.

3 refresher level

For riders returning after a long break who want to ride four or five days a week, who want to ride a century (100 miles/160 km), and who want to start riding with a club.

4 intermediate level

For regular riders cycling for an hour or more four to six times a week, who want to train for a first racing performance.

5 expert level 1

For experienced riders (categories, or "Cats," 4-2) training five or six times a week, who want to set and achieve new personal goals.

6 expert level 2

For experienced riders (Cats 2 and 1) training about 20 hours a week for high level performances.

get things rolling

By now you probably can't wait to get out on the road. But before you head to the garage to drag out that dusty old shopping bike, here are two things you must do first:

check your health

You probably have a reasonable idea of your level of fitness. Are you a sports fanatic, a couch potato, or somewhere in between? As a precaution, see your doctor before starting any new physical activity. Ask him or her to give you a general check-up and advise you on whether there's any condition you have that might mean you should take things slowly.

make sure you can ride

It may sound silly, but the last thing you want is to head off and then realize you can't remember how to brake or change gear, or can't balance properly. If this sounds familiar, take

do you want a race?

There's no unwritten law of cycling that says you must race—it's enough that you enjoy your riding when you do it. But at some point you're probably going to want to try racing, out of curiosity if nothing else. Regular racing also offers you a fixed goal to work toward, a chance to raise your fitness to new heights, and a real sense of achievement once you've crossed that finish line.

your bike to a grassy area and reacquaint yourself with the basic skills and feel of riding before braving the traffic. If you feel that you need more than this, some local community centers, schools, and even bike stores run cycling proficiency courses to help you get to grips with the basic skills and rules of the road.

Even if you're already an experienced cyclist, if you haven't ridden for about a year it's worth completing both of the stages above before you ease back into training, using the specially designed refresher course (see pp. 66–69).

go clubbing

If you want to get the most out of your riding, find a club. Some clubs run beginners' sessions, and usually take on riders of varying abilities. Your local bicycle store should have details of your local clubs and where they meet, or you can find an online list of clubs at the web site of the governing body for road cycling, the United States Cycling Federation (USCF), *www.usacycling.org.*

who do you race?

The USCF categorizes road racers in levels 1 to 5 (Cat 1 for the best amateurs, Cat 5 for novice racers), and Cats 1 to 4 for women. Everyone starts out as a Cat 5 (or Cat 4), and you move up the ranks as you place higher in events. There are also age categories (30+ Masters, 50+ Masters, and so on), which are often filled with experienced older riders.

do you need a club?

You can race without joining a club, but you will need a USCF license ($45 for a year, though you can get one-day versions). To find races in your area, ask at your local bike store, contact the USCF, or visit a listings site on the internet, such as that at *www.bicycling.com.*

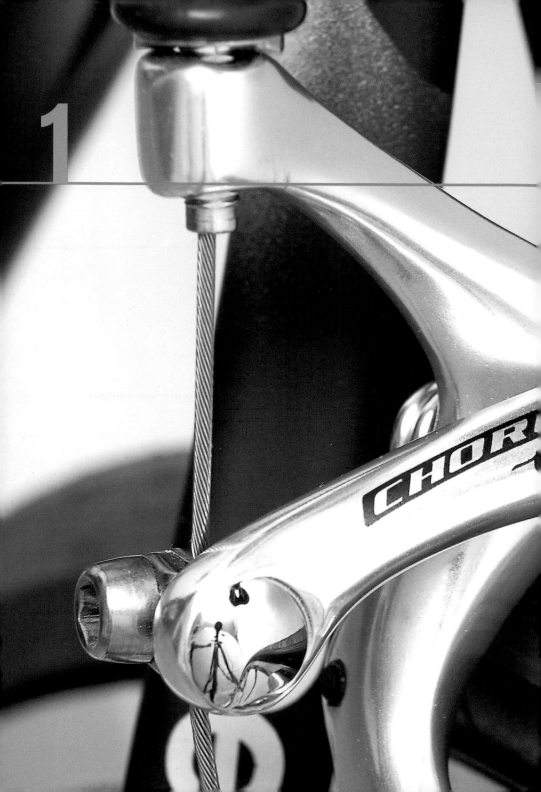

all kitted out

To get the most out of your cycling, you need to do more than just ride. The right bike, the right clothes, the right food—all of these things will make your riding experiences much more enjoyable, your training more productive, and your racing more competitive.

In the following chapter you'll learn more about your bike and the equipment you'll need for comfortable year-round riding. You'll discover what to eat to boost your health and performance, and how to avoid injuries. There are also tips on keeping your enthusiasm riding high, whatever happens.

cycle surgery

R ide, steed, wheels—whatever you call it, the right bike is essential for great cycling. There are many different styles of bike, from tandems (for two people) and hybrids (the traditional "shopping bike") to full suspension mountain bikes and recumbents (seated bicycles). For all-around fitness and competitive road riding, the best type of bike is the racer. Opposite are the things you should look out for when buying one.

pedal power

"DO I REALLY NEED special pedals?" is a question new riders often ask. Although you can ride very well with simple flat pedals or the toe-clips and straps used by riders up to the 1980s, clipless pedals make pedaling more efficient (because the foot and pedal act as one unit to generate power through a much larger part of the pedal circle than simply pushing on a flat pedal) and make the foot more secure when balancing, cornering, or pushing hard while out of the saddle.

saddle ▶▶

Road saddles often look extremely uncomfortable to the novice. But in the last ten years, saddle design has improved to combine the very best compact cushioning to help absorb shock.

wheels ▶▶

Light, spoked wheels with narrow rims and smooth tires are aerodynamic, and are easy to get moving and keep rolling, because they create little friction with the road.

tires ▶▶

Most road bikes use tires with a separate inner tube and are known as clinchers.

chain set ▶▶

Divided into five parts—cranks, chain rings, chain, sprockets (or cassette), and derailleurs—the chain set is the most complicated mechanical part of your bike. Here, leg power is converted into rear wheel motion.

▼ stem

The length of the stem will adjust your riding position on the bike. If the stem is too long, you will be too stretched out; if it is too short, you will be forced to ride hunched up.

◄◄ handlebars

Make sure they are roughly the same width as your shoulders. Ride with your hands on the cross bar or brake hoods (at the end of the cross bar) for comfort, and only use the lowest handlebars (the drops) for hard cycling and extra control on descents and corners.

◄◄ brake and gear levers

These are integrated into one unit (the hoods) on most modern road bikes. Squeeze the levers toward you to brake, push them across toward the front wheel to change gear.

◄◄ headset

Simply put, the tighter your headset (the ball bearings upon which the steering axis rotates), the less your handlebars will turn. Get an experienced mechanic to show you how to adjust the tightness so that it is snug but not locked solid.

▲ frame

Steel, aluminum, titanium, even carbon fiber. Road bike frames are light, nimble, and stiff (so the frame transmits maximum power from the pedals to the rear wheel, which would be partially lost if the frame could bend), but are also designed to absorb the vibrations of the road.

◄◄ brakes

Good-quality brakes are precisely built mechanisms that allow you to modulate brake pressure. The pads should be positioned close to the wheel rim and changed regularly for good braking in all weather conditions.

get wheels

Now that you know the basic parts of a bike, it's time to buy one. The best place to buy a quality road bike is from a specialist. You can buy from large department stores, mail order, the internet, and even private, secondhand dealers, but it's not a good idea for your first buy.

You need a bike that is the right size for you. A road cycling store should be able to measure you and fit you to the best frame and bike for your needs (ask the store to write down the information for future reference). If it is not willing to take your measurements or discuss what kind of bike you're looking for, walk away and go somewhere else.

what to look for

It's a good idea to decide on your budget before you start shopping. The store will try to sell you as many things as it can (it's business after all), but $700 to $900 should buy you a good quality bike. Here are some useful tips to help you choose:

■ Ask about store-soiled frames, or last season clearance purchases. These are often just as good as brand new frames (provided you don't mind the occasional scratch in the paintwork), and because

keep it clean

1 Clean the whole bike (do it regularly with a smooth, damp cloth and then a smooth, dry cloth). Make sure you get into the area behind the cranks and between the brake parts.

2 Clean the chain and all the parts it comes into contact with (chain rings, cassette, and rear derailleur flywheels) using a cloth and cleaning fluid. Use an old toothbrush to clean in any small gaps.

3 Rinse the cleaning fluid off with water and dry thoroughly with a smooth cloth.

4 Use a basic lubricant like WD40 to force any remaining water out of crevices and dry again thoroughly.

5 Oil the chain and derailleurs using a high-quality chain lubricant. Take care not to drip any oil on the braking surfaces of your wheels. Also check tire pressures weekly—underinflated tires can be a safety hazard.

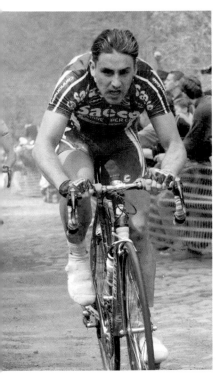

fine-tuning your position

Once you've purchased your bike, you need to find the most comfortable riding position. Once again, ask the experts at your bike store for help, and remember that the most important factor is feel. If your bike doesn't feel comfortable, you're not going to want to ride it. Your store should be able to determine the best riding position for you when it measures you for your bike. There are two main problem areas—get someone to hold the bike while you sit on it and perform these tests:

SADDLE HEIGHT

Remove your shoes and sit on your bike with your hands on the drops. Place one of your heels on a pedal and fully extend your leg. Your leg should be straight when the crank is in line with the seat tube of the frame. If your leg is bent, raise your saddle. If your heel cannot reach the pedal, drop your saddle until it can.

SADDLE POSITION

If your saddle is too far back, you will overstretch to reach the handlebars, and it will be difficult to apply full pressure on the pedals.

Put your bike shoes on, and turn the pedals until the cranks are parallel to the floor. Drop a plumb line from the outside of your knee. The line should hang in line with the middle of your shoe cleat and the pedal axle. Move the saddle forward and back until it does so.

they are store soiled, will be cheaper and therefore better value for your money.

■ Get the right size frame. It's better to have a small frame with a long stem, high seat, and raised headset, than a frame that is simply too big.

maintenance

It's best to leave the more complicated jobs to the mechanics at your bike shop—at least initially. The only job you need to do regularly (say once every one or two weeks) is clean and oil the gears (see box opposite).

summer holidays

You can quite happily ride around in any old clothes you choose. But proper cycling gear is comfortable, practical, and looks good, too. You'll also feel good, which will increase your desire to ride.

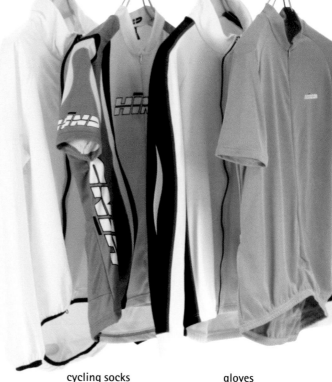

waterproof

There's always the possibility of a sudden downpour when you're out on the road, so carry a lightweight, breathable waterproof rolled up in one of your jersey pockets to stay dry.

jersey

Any lightweight, sweat-wicking T-shirt will be adequate for cycling, but a proper short-sleeved cycle jersey will fit snugly and the pockets on the lower back are surprisingly large and very useful. You can also buy sleeveless versions for those really scorching days. (But don't forget your sunscreen!)

cycling socks

Made of wicking materials to keep your feet sweat-free, specialized "technical" socks are comfortable and have a low-cut cuff to prevent them from catching on your chain.

gloves

Even in hot weather, fingerless cycling gloves are a good idea. They cushion your hands against the vibrations from the road, and protect them in the unlikely event that you fall off.

Warm-weather cycling requires clothing that is snug without being constricting (so it won't flap about as you ride), and fabrics that are light, breathable, and don't saturate with sweat (unlike cotton). Long zips on jerseys are also a particularly good option in case you get really hot and need to pull the zipper down to your waist.

cycling shorts
Stretch fit, padded cycle shorts are very comfortable for riders of both sexes. For a more secure fit, consider bib shorts. These have built in lycra braces, and won't slip down your butt as you ride.

sports bra
A vital part of kit for all women, regardless of bust size. Sports bras reduce breast movement by about 25 percent more than everyday bras.

winter warmers

Despite the threat of wind, rain, and cold, you'll probably find that you still want to ride during the winter. And if you cover up in clothing of the type listed below, go ahead.

A winter kit needs to be windproof and reasonably waterproof to keep out any sudden cold downpours of rain. You don't want to overdress, but it's a good idea to carry an extra layer in case you get really cold. Fabrics that don't get cold when they are wet (such as some specialized "technical" wool mixes) are especially useful.

tips for winter clothing

1 get windproof
You're moving at quite a speed on a bike, which increases the wind chill significantly. Windproof materials such as Gore-Tex will act as a barrier to the wind, keeping you much warmer. Layering your clothes will also help by trapping several layers of warm air as further insulation.

2 wear less, carry extra
Before you start moving, you should feel slightly cool. Once you get moving, your heart rate and body temperature will rise, and it is possible to overheat even on the coldest days. But still carry a spare layer (such as a gilet) in case the temperature drops.

3 cover your extremities
Hands, feet, head, and particularly ears suffer the most in cold weather, so make sure they are well covered before you head out.

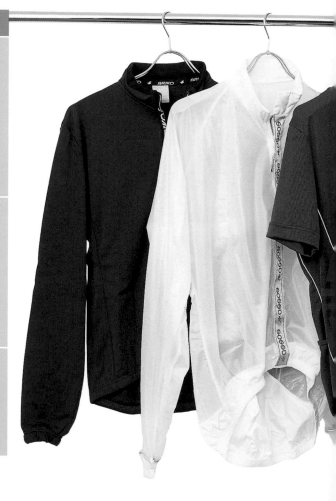

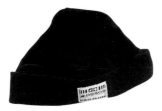

winter gloves
Hands, like feet, get cold quickly on a bike, and numb fingers don't brake or change gear well. Good winter gloves will keep your hands warm and dry, but are flexible enough to change gear and brake without much loss of touch.

hat
A thin, close-fitting beanie hat is ideal for wearing under your cycle helmet on really cold days. Find one that comes down over your ears if necessary.

long–sleeve top
This can be a long-sleeve jersey, or a base layer similar to that worn for skiing. Put it on under you summer jersey.

arm and leg warmers
Another great standby. Arm and leg warmers are simple spandex tubes designed to be slid on at a moment's notice to prevent a chill.

gilet
A gilet is a lightweight sleeveless jacket that often doubles as a waterproof. A great standby to stuff into a jersey pocket.

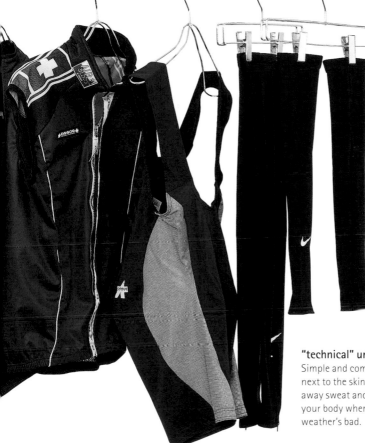

overshoes
Neoprene overshoes are invaluable. Your feet don't flex much when cycling and get cold quickly. Overshoes will keep heat in and the rain out, which makes for a much more comfortable ride.

tights
The winter tights worn by joggers can easily be worn under or over your normal cycling shorts. But for maximum warmth, full-length bib tights with built in windproof panels are a worthwhile buy.

"technical" undershirt
Simple and comfortable next to the skin. It wicks away sweat and warms your body when the weather's bad.

cycling accessories

Cycling offers a myriad of different ways to spend money—there's always a new gadget on the market. Some of these gadgets are more useful than others. Some are vital, such as waterbottles, puncture repair kits, and pumps. Some are very useful, such as cycle computers and heart rate monitors. Some are just a waste of cash—you decide what these are.

helmet ▸▸

Cycling helmets are not a legal requirement, but they are certainly a good idea. Your helmet should fit snugly, and should be worn across the brow, not tipped onto the back of the head.

◂◂ bike shoes

As we have seen, clipless pedals are far more efficient than flat pedals or toe-clips. Special shoes like these have cleats mounted into the sole that then clip into the pedals (the cleats should be positioned in the middle of the ball of the foot). The sole should also be stiff for maximum power transfer.

sunglasses ▸▸

Bright sunlight is wonderful, unless you're trying to pick your way along a twisty road with it shining in your eyes. Standard UV-protection sunglasses are adequate, but make sure they won't fall off as you ride.

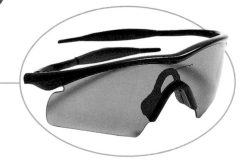

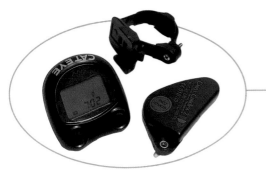

◄◄ cycle computer

A good buy in a little package. An on-board computer lets you monitor your current, average, and maximum speed, distance traveled, and time elapsed. Some can record your cadence (pedal revolutions per minute) and tell you what gear you're in.

heart rate monitor ►►

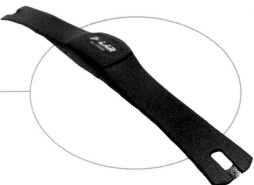

Perhaps the most useful training tool on the market. A strap that fits across your chest reads your heart rate and relays the reading to a wristwatch. By calculating your heart rate (see pp. 40–41) you can keep track of the intensity of your training in a very precise way. There are even models that can calculate your training zones for you.

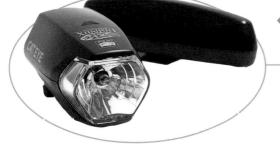

◄◄ lights

Essential if you're riding in the dark, but also useful in rain and mist. A flashing red LED is ideal for the rear, but on the front you need a strong beam halogen powered by a battery that fits into one of your bottle cages, so that it lasts a long time.

pump ►►

A light pump that attaches to the frame of your bike is essential; otherwise when you get a puncture, you're going to be faced with a long walk home.

fuel story

One of the best things about getting involved in a sport like cycling is the food! Unlike many sports, cycling is an activity that you can comfortably sustain for hours, making it ideal for burning the calories provided by food. This is an excellent reason to eat (healthily, of course). In this section, you'll find everything you need to know about eating for cycling, from general information about healthy eating habits to how much to eat to when best to eat for maximum performance.

the food groups

carbohydrates

Carbohydrates (carbs) provide the energy to cycle. They come in two forms: simple carbs (such as sugars) and complex carbs (most starches). A healthy diet should contain both types. Your body absorbs different types of carbs, from different sources, at different speeds. The smaller the carbohydrate food particle, the greater the percentage of water it contains, the lower its protein, fat, and fiber content, and the faster it is absorbed.

Fast-absorbing foods include sports drinks, bananas, sugars, potatoes, and breads. Foods that are absorbed more slowly (and are better suited to providing sustained energy) include oats, pasta, basmati rice, and beans. Make carbohydrates around 65 percent of your daily diet.

water

Water is absolutely critical—lack of water will kill us long before lack of food. Aim to drink about eight glasses of water per day, plus an extra one for every half hour you spend exercising.

protein

Protein provides our bodies with the resources to rebuild itself after strenuous exercise. Without it, our muscles and tendons struggle to keep up with our increased activity. The best sources of protein are meat, poultry, and fish, but nuts, grains, beans, and dairy products are also good, too. Protein can take a long time to be absorbed by your body, so it is best eaten regularly in small quantities with every meal. Aim to make protein around 20 percent of your daily diet.

You need to bear in mind that everyone is different. Different genders, metabolic rates, and levels of exercise intensity mean everyone needs different quantities of each of the food groups.

Use the formula on page 27 to calculate your dietary needs, then apply the percentages given.

A high-energy gel provides a good performance boost.

fat

Fat has had a bad press in recent years, but it is a vital source of energy. It is also used to provide a layer of protective cells around internal organs and to transport fat-soluble vitamins in the bloodstream.

However, too much of the wrong sorts of fat, usually referred to as saturated fat (found in red meat and dairy products), can cause health problems. Good fats are known as mono- and polyunsaturated fats, and can be found in olive oil, nuts, avocados, and oily fish. Aim to make mono- and polyunsaturated fats 25 percent of your diet.

healthy eating

1 fruit and vegetables

Eat more than five portions of fruit and vegetables per day (try to aim for four or five of each).

2 water

Drink a glass of water every morning when you get up, with every meal, and every evening before bed. Carry a bottle around with you as well.

3 protein

Eat a small portion of quality protein with every meal

4 low fat

Eat low-fat dairy products every day (lower fat dairy products actually provide more vitamins and minerals per fluid ounce than full fat ones).

5 iron

Consider an iron supplement, particularly if you're a vegetarian or don't eat red meat.

feeding times

When we cycle, our energy needs are supplied by a combination of carbohydrates, stored as a substance called glycogen, and fat. The body's fat stores are almost always large enough to provide their share, but it's surprisingly easy to run low on glycogen. For maximum performance, keep your carbohydrate reserves high.

how much do I need to eat?

The actual amount of food you need in a day depends on several things:

SEX (basal rate)
Men—11 calories per pound (24 calories per kilogram) of bodyweight.
Women—10 calories per pound (22 calories per kilogram) of bodyweight.

LIFESTYLE
Add an additional 30 to 40 percent for a sedentary job, such as office work.
Add an additional 50 to 60 percent for an active job, such as construction work.

EXERCISE
Add 400 calories per hour of steady cycling.
Add 600 calories per hour of hard cycling.

SO...
A 130 lb (60 kg) female office worker who rides steadily for one hour per day will need:
130 lb x 10 = 1300 + (35% x 1300) = 1755 + 400 = 2155 calories per day.

HOW TO EAT:

WELL BEFOREHAND
It can take between 12 and 24 hours for food to be fully digested by the body. Eat balanced meals the lunchtime and evening before a long or hard morning ride (or evening and breakfast before an evening ride). Regular feeding will keep your glycogen stores steady, so all you need to do before getting on your bike is build them up (see below).

JUST BEFOREHAND
Foods like pasta, muesli, and rye bread release their energy slowly and steadily. Eat them one hour before you ride for sustained energy during training.

KEEP EATING
You will need to refuel in the saddle during any ride lasting more than an hour. Sports drinks, energy gels, and bars are ideal (see pp. 28–29), but raisins, jellybeans, hard candies, and jelly sandwiches will also work. Start refueling 15 minutes into a long ride.

DRINK UP
Most people do not drink enough water. You need to be hydrated to get the most out of your riding. That means sipping water throughout the day, drinking at least 1 pint (500–750 ml) about 30 minutes before you ride, sipping water (or a sports drink) every 15 minutes during your ride, and, afterwards, drinking 1 pint (500–750 ml) for every pound (0.5 kg) of bodyweight you have lost during your ride. Carry your drinks in a water bottle in a bottle cage on your bike.

EAT AFTERWARD

Your body needs replacement energy and protein to recover after a ride. Try to eat within an hour of finishing your ride. Have a tuna salad sandwich, a rice and bean salad, or a bowl of cereal with a banana and a low-fat yogurt.

how to manage your weight

Effective long-term weight loss requires patience. The simple formula is: eat about 500 calories per day less than your need. Or simply eat slightly less and exercise more. The key is to stick with your plan. Try these techniques:

1 Commit to regular exercise. Get out on your bike and ride as often as possible.

2 Make small changes to your diet. Be realistic. Do you have a "problem" food? Try to find a healthier alternative (for example, frozen yogurt or sorbet instead of ice cream) and eat smaller portions.

3 Graze. Eat frequent small meals to burn more calories; just make sure the meals are healthy.

4 Plan your meals. If you know what you're going to eat and when, you're less likely to stray.

5 Count portions, not calories. Calorie counting is often obsessive and depressing. Think in terms of fist-sized portions instead.

6 Load up on vegetables. Vegetables are low in calories, but high in nutrition. Make them a part of every meal.

food on the move

We've already seen that constant refueling is vital on long rides (see pp. 26–27). The further you go, the more important it becomes to carry extra fuel. But what should you eat, how much, and when?

what?

There are two types of mid-ride food. Bananas, diluted fruit juice, pretzels, jelly sandwiches, and candies are used to great effect by many cyclists. But other people will find that these are difficult to eat while cycling, or that these simply don't provide the energy that they require.

Avoid fatty or high-protein foods during rides—they take too long to digest.

A more technical approach is to use the special sports drinks and food products available. Sports drinks (which usually come as a powder), and energy gels or bars, are easily absorbed by the body for quick, but sustained, energy. Look for ones that contain electrolytes (see panel) and include glucose polymers or maltodextrin for energy (but it is important to remember to drink water every time you eat a gel or bar).

Different things work for different people, so experiment with your intake until you find a combination of foods and drink you enjoy and can stomach.

how much?

Your body can absorb between 250 and 400 calories per hour. That's the equivalent of two pints (one liter) of most sports drinks, one large energy bar, or five large bananas.

when?

Ideally you should eat and drink at regular intervals of about 15 minutes when you're riding. In practice, this isn't always possible. Here are three tips:

- Start eating early—take your first mouthful of drink as you get underway, and have your first solids after about 20 minutes.

- Eat when the pace slows—on fast group rides or in races grab this opportunity to eat and drink.

- Eat on descents—refueling while climbing is not usually possible, so start to make up the deficit as soon as you're over the top of the hill. Just be careful on those downhill corners!

On most long rides, your body should be able to absorb both solids and liquids without difficulty. As you start racing, however, you may find that your stomach cannot cope with solid foods. If so, use a sports drink that can be safely mixed to higher concentrations.

bonk—that hurt!

Experienced cyclists will know the perils of the "bonk" or "hunger knock." This is a state that results from failure to refuel sufficiently during hard rides. Much like hitting the "wall" in a marathon, the bonk means that your body has run out of available carb-based energy and is having to burn more fat instead. More oxygen is required to burn fat compared to carbohydrates, so your breathing and heart rate increase and you have to work much harder to maintain your pace. The bonk is unpleasant, so be sure to refuel properly at all times.

a pinch of salts

There's one other important part of mid-ride nutrition—electrolytes. Without minerals such as sodium and potassium, the body will not become thirsty or absorb water, which can lead to bloating and, even worse, dehydration, nausea, and vomiting. Make sure that your sports drink contains electrolytes.

chain reactions

Performing well as a cyclist requires a certain amount of determination to push yourself to new limits. However, novices often try to push too far, too hard. This invariably leads to injury and exhaustion.

injury

Injury is almost always pain specific, meaning that the spot that hurts is the injured area. If your knee feels sore and painful as your ride, you've probably injured it. If a specific pain appears, stop and rest for a minute. Then get on your bike and spin (cycle in a low gear) very gently. If the pain doesn't reappear, gradually pick up the pace. If it still does not return, it's probably safe to restart your session. If the pain does return, spin home slowly and

accident and recovery

CRASHING

There's always a possibility that you might be unlucky and crash. In the worst cases this can lead to a trip to a hospital, but more usually it results in bruises, shock, and a lot of raw skin from skidding along the road. If you are in any doubt about how you feel after a crash, go to a hospital.

If you are certain this isn't necessary, walk or get a lift home, and take the next day or two off training. Your body will probably be sore and stiff. Keep all cuts clean, and change any dressings regularly. Use the R.I.C.E procedure opposite to remedy any bad bruising.

R.I.C.E

R–rest
Stop training until the injury has healed, and try to keep your weight off the injured area.

I–ice
Firmly apply an ice pack (or a bag of frozen peas) wrapped in a towel to the injured area. Alternatively, give yourself an ice massage, rubbing the injured area with an ice cube. Do either of these for 15 minutes every hour, or as often as you can manage, to reduce inflammation.

C–compression
Bandage the area firmly (but not so that it restricts the circulation) to reduce inflammation. Anti-inflammatory drugs such as ibuprofen can also help.

E–elevation
In the early stages of recovery, raise the injured area to reduce the quantity of blood flowing to it. This will help minimize tissue damage.

apply R.I.C.E. (see below). If the injury persists see your doctor, or better still, a sports medicine specialist.

overtraining

It's easy to get overenthusiastic about cycling, and if you're not careful you could end up overtrained (or more accurately, under-recovered). Symptoms of overtraining include general lethargy, a high resting heart rate (see pp. 40–41), loss of appetite (or sudden changes in appetite), weight loss, constant colds, and an inability to lift your heart rate while riding. If so, think back. Have you been taking enough rest days? Are you constantly trying to push harder? Are you eating properly? Take a couple of days off training, and then gently ease back in. Monitor closely how you feel and do not try to push through it—your body is telling you to stop. You will only end up feeling worse, or injuring yourself.

train wisely

GET WELL SOONER

Everyone gets ill occasionally. When it happens, perform this simple analysis:

■ Are the symptoms confined to my head? Stuffy noses and mild headaches can be ridden through, but don't do any hard riding. If your symptoms have spread elsewhere (upset stomach, wheezing, fever), don't ride at all until they have passed.

■ Am I well enough to work? Be realistic. If you are too ill to go to work, you are too ill to cycle. (This applies even if you're going to work anyway!)

Take at least one total rest day every week. Check your heart rate before you get out of bed in the morning. Get to know what it should be, and if the rate is more than five beats above normal when you wake, take an extra day's rest.

motive and opportunity

We all have bad days. Sometimes the last thing you want to do is get on your bike. This is only natural, and a few missed days are nothing to worry about. But you don't want to lose your enthusiasm completely, so it's good to have a few ways of keeping your motivation levels high.

set a goal

Having a target to work toward is a great way to stay focused. Just make sure it is a realistic one. If you're a new

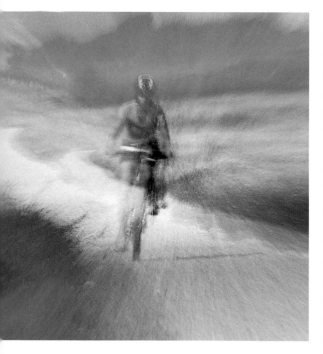

rider, your goal should be one hour's non-stop riding. If you are more experienced, consider building up to a century (100-mile/160-km) ride or really test your fitness in a 10-mile (16-km) time trial.

think big

At the start of each year, plan what you want to get out of your riding. Whether it's losing some weight or completing a particular race distance, know where you are going.

think small

Once you know your endpoint, break your task down into small, manageable pieces. Set yourself a monthly goal (a short race or a speed test—see p. 65), and select a particular session you want to do well each week.

enjoy

This is an essential element, particularly for beginners. You should be riding first and foremost because you enjoy it. If you start to lose that feeling, forget your pre-planned sessions and just ride for the fun of it. Go as far as you like and as fast or slow as you like. Stop for coffee and cake. It doesn't matter. Just enjoy it.

beating the blues

Here are some ways to combat specific motivation problems:

1

Problem:
"I've been riding every day and it's getting boring."

Solution:
Take a week off and do something else to keep active.

2

Problem:
"I'm lonely cycling on my own."

Solution:
Join a club and find a whole new group of friends to ride with.

3

Problem:
"Everyone is faster than me."

Solution:
Ignore them. Focus on your own improvements.

4

Problem:
"Cycling doesn't seem novel any more."

Solution:
Buy some new accessories. There's nothing like having new toys to play with.

5

Problem:
"I'm too busy at work."

Solution:
Commute by bike. It's great exercise and kind to the environment.

Keep a diary of your riding. Use it to plan your sessions, record your times and feelings, and chart your improvements. A look through your diary should remind you of your goals and motivate you by showing you just how much you have improved.

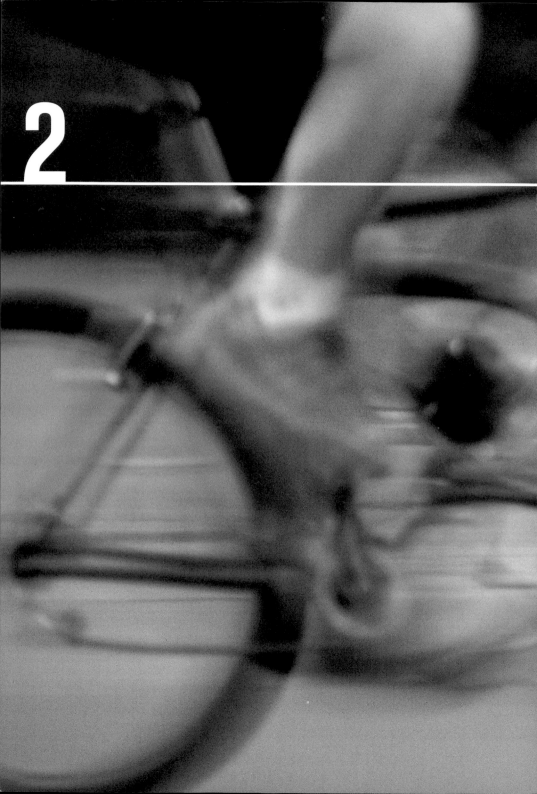

2

training schedules

Cyclists agree that one of the best ways to improve is to follow a specific training schedule. If this sounds too much like hard work, take heart. You don't have to commit to any more than you want to. The biggest benefit of a training schedule is that it gives structure to your week and provides a series of goals to aim for. You'll also have the satisfaction of knowing that you've achieved something new after you've completed each schedule.

In this chapter, you'll learn the different training techniques, learn the technical cycling skills, and follow training schedules that will take you from beginner to experienced racing cyclist.

finding your level

Training is usually only associated with the fastest, strongest, and most competitive cyclists. The truth is, of course, that every time you go out for a bike ride you are training. All training really involves is increasing your fitness. In this chapter, you'll find training to suit two types of rider. Goal-oriented riders will find training schedules that are targeted at specific objectives, from riding for one hour to racing.

Riders who do not feel the need for a specific goal, or who are facing a long winter break without racing, will find a series of four-week schedules, designed to be repeated, to keep them

which schedule is for you?

1 starter level 1	**2** starter level 2	**3** refresher level
pages 60–61	**pages 62–65**	**pages 66–69**
For: Complete beginners.	For: Beginners who have a month's experience.	For: New riders looking for a new challenge or experienced riders returning after a break.
Includes: Riding four days a week, gradually increasing your time on the bike.	Includes: Riding four days a week, gradually increasing distance and speed.	Includes: Riding four or five days a week, gradually increasing distance and speed.
Use this schedule for: Building up fitness and experience from nothing.	Use this schedule for: Getting cycling fit for the first time. Preparing yourself before you start riding with a club.	Use this schedule for: Preparing for your first century (100-mile/160-km) ride. Finding your legs when you join a cycle club.

fit without building their fitness to a race-ready peak.

There are also skill masterclasses in climbing, descending, sprinting, cornering, bunch riding, and solo racing (time trials), as well as information on organizing a full year of training, how to train without leaving the house, weight training for cycling, and stretching.

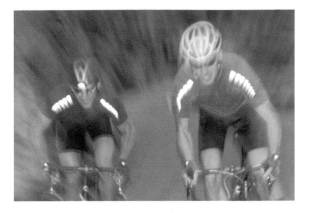

4 intermediate level

pages 70–75

For: Regular club riders (USCF Cats 5 and 4) who want to start racing more regularly.

Includes:
Riding four to six days a week with goal-specific sessions of one hour or more.

Use these schedules for: All-around fitness. Preparing to race a century (100 miles/160 km). Getting started in time trials.

5 expert level 1

pages 76–81

For: Riders with a season of racing experience who want to improve their times.

Includes:
Riding five or six days a week with goal-specific sessions of one hour or more.

Use these schedules for: All-around fitness. Racing criteriums (see pp. 80–81). Road events. Improving your time trialing.

6 expert level 2

pages 82–87

For: Riders with several seasons racing experience who want to make the most of their abilities.

Includes:
Riding five or six days a week, and up to 20 hours in the saddle.

Use these schedules for: All-around fitness. Racing at the front in criteriums and road events. Breaking the hour mark for a 25-mile (40-km) time trial.

the cycle of the seasons

You can cycle in almost any weather. It's not uncommon for the same group of riders to be seen out in the scorching heat of summer and braving the iciest roads in winter. That said, there is a definite seasonal quality to racing. In the northern hemisphere, most of the road races and time trials are held in the spring, summer, and early autumn, with only the tough competitors of cyclo-cross (a road and cross-country event) racing during the depths of winter. There is little point, then, in building yourself to peak race fitness in late November. It makes more sense to divide the year up by seasons.

do's and don'ts of training

do
Build fitness slowly—you need time to grow stronger, or you'll end up injured.

do
Take total rest days—you can only build fitness during recovery. Take at least one day off from all riding every week.

do
Be consistent—regular training is the key to improvement.

do
Spin a smaller gear—as a rule, your legs should feel like they are turning slightly too fast (a cadence of about 90 rpm). Only push large gears when your training specifically demands it (see p. 43 and p. 87).

do
Warm-up and cooldown—your body needs to ease into activity. Spin (see left) for about 10 minutes before and after any hard session, and stretch after all training (see pp. 58–59).

don't
Increase your weekly training by more than about 15 percent per week.

don't
Skip training unless you're ill, injured, or overtrained.

what to focus on and when

winter ▶▶

Build your endurance with long, steady rides. Build your strength with weights and, in late winter, train for strength on the bike. Work on your technical skills and focus on any specific weaknesses.

Try a cyclo-cross race for fun and as a hard effort workout, and a steady-paced century ride for quality endurance training.

spring ▶▶

Build your speed endurance and power by focusing more on tempo riding (see p. 43) and begin to build up your speed work (see p. 43). Use early season races to gauge your fitness level.

Try early season time trials to really work on your speed endurance ability.

summer ▶▶

Peak for racing by focusing on speed work. Practice race skills like climbing hard, responding to attacks (where leading riders break away from the bunch), and sprinting when tired. Make sure that, once you start racing, you are recovering fully between events.

Try to beat your best times at your favorite events or at a new challenge, such as a race you haven't done before.

autumn ▶▶

Continue to race and recover until your final target event. Then take one or two weeks rest. Then gradually start again, focusing on endurance and technique.

Try going out in a blaze of glory—build your last weeks of training for an all-out attempt at a best performance. Then take two weeks off to bask in the glory.

hard at work 1

Cycling doesn't have to be hard. You don't have to push yourself all the time. It's enough that you're enjoying your riding and doing it on a regular basis. But sooner or later, you'll want a challenge. Over the next four pages, you'll find out how to measure your pace when riding, how to test yourself to see how much you've improved, as well as discover the different kinds of training you can do to improve your speed.

Heart rate monitors come in two parts: the sensors on the chest strap pick up your pulse, which is then relayed to the wristwatch.

the heart of the matter

A heart rate monitor is an invaluable tool for training. Unlike speed, which can be affected by weather conditions and terrain, you heart rate is the true indicator of physical stress. There are some reasonably priced beginners' models on the market, and they're really very simple to use (see p. 23).

max heart rate

To train effectively, you need to push yourself to your maximum heart rate (MHR), which is measured in beats per minute (bpm). Beginners, or overweight riders (with 20 percent or more body fat) can use the formula below to work out what their maximum heart rate is.

However, the figure you calculate this way is only a guideline. A better way to find your MHR is with a climb test. Only riders who have completed both Starter Levels should consider this (it is very hard work).

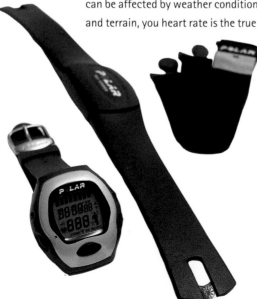

maximum heart rate

MEN: 214 – (0.8 x age)

WOMEN: 209 – (0.9 x age)

So a 30-year-old man would have an MHR of:

0.8 x 30 = 24
Then 214—24 = 190 bpm

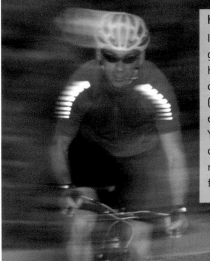

how fast am I?

It's only natural to want to know how fast you can go. It's also useful to know your maximum pace (for hard, consistently fast riding). Once you have completed the Starter Level programs in this chapter (see pp. 60–65), replace one of your Sunday endurance rides with a 10-mile (16-km) time trial. You can do this by yourself, or by participating in a club race. Repeat the same course every couple of months and record your time, speed, heart rate, and feelings about the ride.

Ride slowly for 15 to 60 minutes, arriving at the bottom of a hill that would normally take you 5 to 10 minutes to climb, and is not too steep (no more than a seven percent gradient). Pick a spinning (low) gear and climb as hard as possible until you have to stop. Coast back down to the bottom of the hill and then immediately repeat the climb test.

Keep a check on your heart rate throughout both efforts (some monitors record the maximum reached during a session). You should hit your MHR during the second climb.

training zones

Almost all the training sessions in these schedules will have a suggested heart rate percentage (see pp. 42–43). To calculate these percentages, first take your MHR and subtract your resting heart rate (which you can take just after you wake in the morning, before you get up). So if your MHR is 190 bpm, and your resting rate is 50 bpm, your working heart rate is 140 bpm. If your session suggests you train at 75 percent, calculate 75 percent of 140 (105), and add that to your resting heart rate (105 + 50 = 155). The result is your target heart rate for the session.

Work out all the percentages in advance, and write them in your training diary or commit them to memory so you don't have to search for a calculator to do your math before each session.

hard at work 2

Now that you know how to measure your effort, start thinking about new sessions to improve your fitness. The schedules in this book use a particular set of training sessions, which are:

types of training session

All of these sessions can be flat or hilly (except the recovery ride). Tailor your training to your weaknesses, and the type and terrain of your target races.

SESSION	ACTIVITY	TARGET HEART RATE	FEELING
RECOVERY	Spinning on flat or gentle hills	60 percent	Easy, relaxed
ENDURANCE	Spinning over long distances	65 percent	Comfortable
STEADY	Pace riding at 70–80 rpm	70 percent	Working
TEMPO	Long intervals with short recoveries	75 percent	Pushing
SPEED WORK	Hard intervals with longer recoveries	80–85 percent	Hard/very hard
SPRINTS	Short 15–30 second bursts	Flat out the whole way	
JUMPS	As for Sprints, but a training partner goes first and you have to follow		
STRENGTH	Intervals in a very large gear	Hard on the legs, not the heart	

different types of interval training

The schedules in this book include four main types of interval training (efforts separated by periods of recovery). Each has a different purpose. Only consider speed work once you have completed the first two Starter Levels (see pp. 60–65) and can comfortably ride for an hour every session.

1

TEMPO
These long intervals are designed to increase your leg strength at speed. They are very useful preparation for time trials and for working well at the front of a pack.

WORK
3–5 x 5–15 min at 75 percent heart rate

REST
2–3 min dropping to 60 percent heart rate

2

SPEED WORK
Slightly shorter intervals designed to increase your pace and tolerance for hard riding.

WORK
4–6 x 3–6 min peaking at 80–85 percent heart rate

REST
30–120 seconds (for pace tolerance); same time as effort (for building quality speed)

3

STRENGTH
These intervals are not very hard on the heart and lungs, but they are completed in a large gear (big chain-ring, small sprocket) at 50 to 70 rpm, so they are hard on the legs. They can be done on the flat to build strength for time trialing or up hills to build strength for climbing. Concentrate on pedaling smoothly.

WORK
From 2–4 x 10–15 min to 4–10 x 3–5 min

REST
Up to 10 min for long intervals, 2–3 min for short intervals

4

SPRINTS
These are flat out efforts ridden out of the saddle in a big or small gear. They can be done on the flat, up hills, off a descent, even around corners. Heart rate is unimportant, as the intervals are too short for the heart to respond fully to the effort. Just go as fast as you can.

WORK
4–12 x 15–30 sec flat out

REST
2–5 min dropping down to 60 percent heart rate

skills: upwardly mobile

Climbing is one of the greatest challenges in cycling. The sense of achievement as you reach the summit of a mountain climb is immense. Many cycle races are won and lost here.

how to do it

Efficient pedaling is vital for good riding. Ride seated, select a low gear, and focus on turning the pedals around in a circle—push down, pull the foot back, lift the knee up and forward, slide the foot forward, and push down once more. Breathe evenly at all times.

how hard

Your effort level will rise naturally as you climb, because you're working against gravity. The secret to strong climbing is the ability to ride fast without working too hard. Start climbing at a steady pace and pace yourself to the top. Only accelerate near the top as the gradient decreases,

help! I can't climb

If you're not a strong climber, but want to keep up with a group of stronger riders, there are two things you can do:

 1 Start the climb at the front of the group. Settle into a rhythm you are comfortable with and try to dictate the pace.

2 When you start to feel tired, gradually drift back from the front and let other riders set the pace. Tuck yourself in behind the wheel of the new front man (if he'll let you) and ride behind him ("drafting"). If the pace gets too hard, drop back another wheel and so on until the top.

■ Include a climb in every ride you do.

■ Increase your leg strength with weight training in the winter.

■ Do tempo sessions on a long, gradual climb to improve your aerobic capacity.

■ Do short strength intervals up sections of a moderate climb. Accelerate for the last minute of the ride if you can.

■ Practice alternating seated and standing climbing positions. Keep pedaling smoothly as you stand up. Many riders stop pedaling for a moment when they rise out of the saddle and lose precious momentum.

and over the crest. Start the climb too hard or in too high a gear and you will quickly become exhausted.

how to do it better

Remain seated as much as possible (you'll use less energy), but shift your position forward and back on the saddle occasionally to work different muscles. To increase your pace, rise out of the saddle and "dance" on the pedals, swaying your body and bike slightly from side to side, and adding your bodyweight to your smooth pedaling.

how hilly? a rough guide to describing a route

1	**flat:** nothing more than the slightest bumps
2	**false flat:** a very slight incline
3	**undulating:** short rises, nothing long or steep
4	**rolling:** regular rises with similar descents. Often short but quite steep.
5	**lumpy:** lots of short, steep climbs and descents
6	**hilly:** climbs of 1–4 miles (1.5–6 km)
7	**mountainous:** climbs of over 4 miles (6 km)

skills: coming down

Flying down a descent is an exhilarating experience. You travel effortlessly at speeds of up to 40 mph (64 km/h). Descents are also one of the most technical aspects of cycling. The potential for injury if you fall also makes it probably the most dangerous.

how to do it

Descending well is about anticipation. Look down the road well ahead of where you're going. Watch for potholes and gravel, and anticipate braking points well before corners. Shift into a higher gear and move your hands onto the drops, resting one or two fingers on the sides of the brake levers. Move your butt to the rear of the saddle to increase the stability of your bike.

On bumpy roads, turn your pedals until the cranks are parallel to the ground and lift yourself up until you hover just above the saddle. Grip the top tube of the frame with your knees to increase stability.

how hard

Descents are an ideal place to recover from the rigors of climbing. Momentum and gravity will pull you down, so all you need to do is turn your legs around gently to keep the muscles loose. Make sure you shift gear if the descent flattens out or rears back up into a climb.

how to do it better

Once you've mastered the basics and are confident descending, there are two techniques you can learn to improve. On long, straight downhills, adopt an aerodynamic "tuck" position. Place your hands close together on the cross bar and rise slightly off the saddle (as you would on a bumpy road). Bend at the waist to bring your head down

Descending is dangerous, but addictive. Always wear a helmet, and try not to take too many risks, particularly during endurance rides.

help! I can't descend

Some riders find descending terrifying. But it's possible to go down fast without losing control.

1 Find a rider who you know descends well and sit three or four bike lengths behind him or her for the descent. Follow the line he or she takes through the corners.

2 Relax your muscles so that you respond more smoothly to corners, steeper sections, and changes in road surface.

close to your hands, so that the wind flows over your back.

The other technique is to use your chest as a parachute to control your pace, rather than your brakes. On long downhills, braking too frequently can cause the brakes and rims to overheat, which can reduce the effectiveness of the brakes.

cornering downhill

Corners on descents are often high speed and high risk. Keep your weight over your back wheel, and shed some speed by braking gently well before the corner. Also avoid speeding down hills in wet, foggy, or windy conditions. It simply isn't worth the risk.

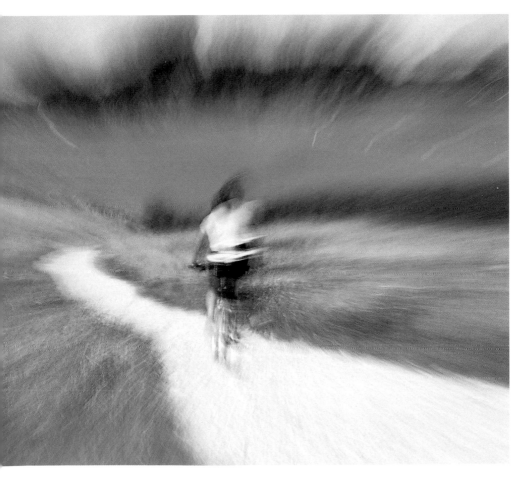

skills: driving around the bend

Two of the most important skills for a competitive rider are sprinting and cornering. The ability to carry speed through corners and sprint out of them is particularly important for the tight circuits around the multilap criterium courses (see pp. 80–81).

The final touch in a sprint finish is to thrust your bike across the line as you sit down. This gives you a final push of forward momentum to carry you across the line.

how to corner

The skills for cornering are much like those for descending. You need to plan your line through the corner and cut as close to the curb as you dare.

■ Corner with your hands on the drops.
■ Look through the corner and quickly plan where you want to end up.
■ Push down lightly on the bars with the hand leading you into the turn.
■ Straighten your outside leg and press your foot onto the pedal.
■ Press into the top tube with your inside knee.

how to corner better

Shift your weight back in the saddle by moving your butt back and keeping

help! I can't corner

If you're struggling with your cornering, there are two things you can do:

 1 Take the "racing line" through the corner. Enter the corner from farther toward the center of the road, and follow a line that takes you close to the curb on the apex of the turn— you'll go through faster. Or simply follow the wheel of the rider ahead.

2 Don't brake or steer. Keep your weight balanced and let your speed carry you through.

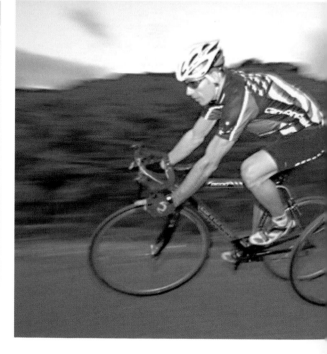

your body low. As you approach the corner, twitch your bike away from the turn very slightly, then steer it back in for a steeper angle as you turn through the corner.

how to sprint

Shift up one gear and jump out of the saddle with your hands on the drops and begin pedaling hard. Shift gears as soon as you begin to feel that you're spinning. Keep your weight back over the back wheel, and pull up with each hand as you push down on the pedals with each foot, but don't fully straighten your legs as you

help! I can't sprint

If you're struggling with your sprinting, there are two things you can do:

1 Follow the wheel of a better sprinter and then try to blast past at the last possible moment.

2 Start to push a lot earlier. Lift the pace as if you were riding the final miles of a time trial and hope your opponents won't be able to hang on.

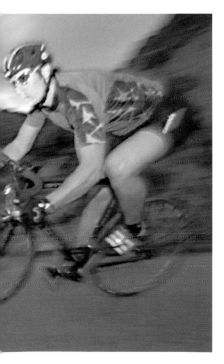

pedal. Keep your head low, but keep looking forward. When you reach your top speed, sit back down, and concentrate on turning the pedals as fast as possible. Don't hold your breath—your body needs all the oxygen it can get.

how to train for sprints

- Build your leg strength by doing uphill sprints and weights in the winter.
- Build your sprint speed by doing long sprints of up to 60 seconds with long recoveries.
- Get used to criterium sprinting by doing short 10-second sprints out of corners on steady rides, and by rolling almost to a standstill before each sprint effort.

skills: in the pack

Riding in a large bunch is an essential skill, whether you're going out for a spin with a few friends or competing in a road race. Drafting is also a great way to save energy. Riders can save up to 25 percent of their energy by "hiding" in the pack.

how hard

The beauty of riding in the pack is that it is considerably easier than riding on your own. A small pack of riders will form a "chain gang" or "pace line" where each rider takes a turn working at the front, followed by a recovery period as he or she drifts to the back. The rotation continues with the next person taking the lead, then dropping back, and so on.

how to do it

Align yourself with the back wheel of the rider in front of you and stay right behind it. If you want to remain strong for a sprint or climb later in the race, try to move up on the outside of the bunch, do some work at the front, and then ease back behind the front riders. If you're not used to riding in a pack, it can be very intimidating. If so, ride near the edge of the pack, but still follow the back wheel in front of you.

how to do it better

Sheltering in a pack becomes much harder in a crosswind. One way to combat a crosswind is to form an "echelon." The lead rider rides with the wind hitting one shoulder. The next cyclist rides on the leader's sheltered shoulder, slightly behind. The next rider does the same with the second rider. After his or her turn, the rider at the head of the echelon drops back to the last position and the rotation continues. Do not form echelons more than three or four deep unless riding on closed roads.

how to train for it

Nervous riders can practice bumping shoulders (a common feature of pack riding) with a training partner on a short, flat grass surface.

Start pack riding with easy group rides with your local cycle club. When you're more confident, try a faster group ride.

rules of the road

1 Don't just watch the wheel in front of you. Watch the road ahead as well and keep an eye on what's happening elsewhere in the pack.

2 Try not to overlap the wheel of the rider in front.

3 Follow the same line around corners as the wheel ahead.

4 Be prepared to switch to single file at any time.

5 Learn the hand signals. Most people already know how to indicate a left and right turn by pointing with the relevant arm.

6 Pointing to the ground and drawing a circle means "hole in the road."

7 Holding an open palm facing back, down by your leg, means "slow down."

8 Tucking the arm nearest the sidewalk behind your back means "stationary object on this side."

9 Keep your ears pricked for calls of "oil," "car," "broken glass," and so on from the front. Pass the call down the group verbally.

10 When you cross an intersection with no cars coming call "clear" so riders behind know it is safe to cross.

skills: go it alone

Solo riding is a complete contrast to riding in a pack. There's no shelter, and no rest apart from the occasional descent. But for many, solo rides—and particularly time trials—are the only way to really gauge one's abilities.

how to do it

Solo riding is about two things— sustained speed and good aerodynamics. Riders in time trials often have specially built bikes with "aero" handlebars on which they can rest their forearms for a more aerodynamic position, and similarly aerodynamic wheels. The fastest even wear special aerodynamic helmets, skin-tight racing suits, and even lycra socks over their shoes. Road riders, too, will mimic this position, riding with

help! I can't time trial

Some riders find burying themselves in hard effort for a long period very difficult. Here are two ways to make the best of a lone push:

1 Don't get stuck in one gear. The temptation is to stick to one gear no matter how hilly the course becomes. Concentrate on maintaining the same cadence instead, shifting gears as necessary to keep moving.

2 Choose more hilly courses. You will have to work hard up the rises, but you will also be able to recover and pick up speed on the way down.

how to train for solo riding

There is no secret to riding hard by yourself—it is all about practice. So just get on your bike and ride! On the right are some tips that will help you improve more quickly and avoid some pitfalls.

their hands in the drops or draped loosely over the handlebars, with arms bent, and their bodies tucked close to the frame. Other than body positioning, though, solo riding is all about hard work.

how hard?

Simple—as hard as you can, relative to the distance you want to cover. But use a gear that lets you pedal smoothly. A large gear will feel easier at first, but your legs will tire quickly. Warm-up before every time trial and stretch afterwards (see p. 38 and pp. 58–59).

how to do it better

Work on your concentration. Focus on your belief that you can keep going. Remember rides when you cycled really well. Keep telling yourself to pedal smoothly. Resist the urge to sprint to maintain your pace, and don't let your pace drop even when you start to tire.

1 Take a turn at the front of the bunch during group rides at every opportunity.

2 Do all your quality training (steady rides, tempo, speed work) alone.

3 Concentrate on speed work with short recoveries. You need to keep going when the pace gets tough.

4 Gradually build the distance you cover in the final interval of your weekly speed work until it becomes a mini-time trial. Or ride short mid-week time trials in place of your speed work (many clubs run evening 10-milers [16 km] in the spring and summer).

staying in shape

tip...
Less is more.
Indoor training
places greater
mental and
physical demands
on your body.
Reduce your
planned session to
three-quarters or
two-thirds of your
original plan, and
spend the extra
time stretching
thoroughly.

Cycling is an outdoor activity. It's about the wind in your hair and the sun on your face.

But it can't always be that way. Some days just aren't meant for cycling. Rain. Icy roads. High winds. These are the days to stay inside.

But that doesn't mean that you can't ride. There are three tools you can use to train indoors.

EXERCISE BIKE

It may have a reputation as an impromptu clothes rack, but one with programmable resistance and training sessions is a good investment. Some even have a race program that mimics gear changes. Check that your riding position and pedaling action are as close to your road position as possible.

Best for: Riding in a gym.

ROLLERS

The simplest way to train indoors, rollers consist of three free-rolling cylinders, one of which is under your front wheel. Two more cylinders support the rear wheel. Rollers mimic the resistance of a flat road. Balance your bike on top of the rollers and ride as normal. Just be careful—it can be tricky to balance at first.

Best for: Practicing balance and riding technique.

inside lines

Training alternatives for indoor sessions:

Keep long rides interesting by mixing in technique sets. Do 10 x one-minute spin-ups where you gradually increase your pedaling until you start bouncing on the saddle. Or try pedaling smoothly using only one leg (rest the other foot on a chair next to you). Also try spinning with your eyes closed to enhance your awareness of the feel of fluid pedaling.

Do tempo riding, strength sessions, and speed work just as you would on the road. Try pyramid sessions (with efforts of one, two, three, four, and five minutes, then back down to one, all with one-minute recoveries), or sessions based around loud music to keep your motivation levels high.

Raise your front wheel slightly (use a telephone directory or catalogues) to simulate your climbing position for a whole session. Remember to set the resistance and gear to complement the effect.

INDOOR TRAINER

Also called a turbo trainer, this A-frame clamps on to your rear wheel and holds your bike in position on a rolling cylinder. Many versions have variable resistance to mimic climbs and headwinds, and some even have built-in computers to monitor your speed, cadence, wattage, and calorie burn.

Best for: Hard training if you live in an area with no quiet roads.

OTHER GEAR FOR INDOOR SESSIONS

You will get very hot and sweaty during indoor sessions, so it's worth remembering the following:

- Drink one bottle of water more than normal.

- Use a towel to drape across the top of your bike to protect it from sweat.

- Use a towel to dry yourself during recoveries.

- Use a large electric fan to cool you down.

- You could even consider setting up your indoor trainer in the garage or under an awning on a porch.

the weighting game

Remember to warm up and maintain your leg speed with 15 minutes of easy spinning before and after your session. You could even try riding to and from the gym to save time.

Professional cyclists tend to have muscular legs and slim upper bodies. But they don't neglect their upper body strength. And neither should you. Regular strength work strengthens the bones and joints, and develops more general fitness. Specific weight training during the winter can make you a stronger, faster rider. The following 30-minute weight-training program can be done in place of two recovery rides each week.

squat ▶▶

Stand with your feet shoulder width apart, with dumbbells held by your sides. Keeping your head looking forward and your back straight, bend at the knees until the backs of your thighs are no more than parallel to the floor. Exhale and push back up to the starting position, then repeat.

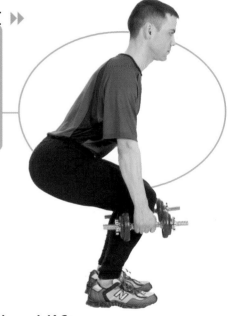

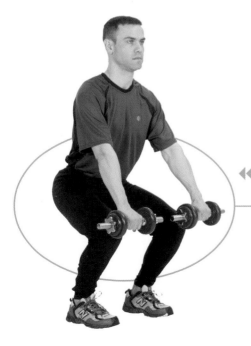

◀◀ dead lift

Stand with your feet shoulder width apart with dumbbells held in front of your thighs (palms facing you). Keeping your arms down and your head looking forward and your back straight, bend at the knees until the backs of your thighs are parallel to the floor. Exhale and push back up, straightening the back, and raising the shoulders slightly as you do so, then repeat.

the most important weights

To train for cycling strength (best done in the winter), concentrate on the squat, dead-lift, bench press, and row. Build these up from three to six sets of eight slow repetitions with a heavy weight. Recover for a full minute between sets.

To train for general fitness, do two to three sets of 12 to 15 repetitions with a moderate weight for all the exercises. Recover for 30 seconds between sets.

bench press ▶▶

Lie on your back with dumbbells held above your chest with straight arms. Inhale and slowly bring the weight down until it touches your chest. Exhale as you push the weight back to the starting position, taking care not to rock or jerk.

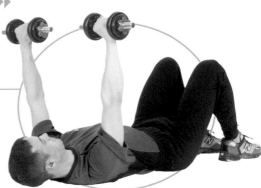

◀◀ row

Bend the knees slightly and bend forward at the waist, keeping the back straight. Let the arms hang to the ground, holding the dumbbell with a wide grip. Pull the weights up by bending the arms until they touch your chest and your elbows point to the ceiling. Then slowly lower and repeat.

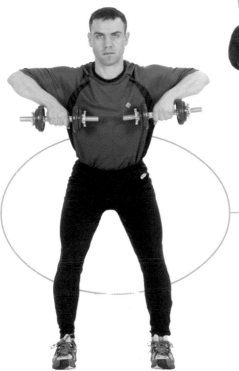

stretch fit

Classes in stretching disciplines, such as yoga and pilates, are great ways of incorporating more complete stretching into your routine. But be careful not to overstretch and injure yourself.

Stiff muscles are more easily damaged, and less responsive when riding, than flexible muscles. You should get into the habit of performing a stretching routine after every ride. The 10-stretch routine below is ideal. Hold each stretch for 30 to 45 seconds, and repeat for each leg. But make sure you don't stretch further than is comfortable.

gastrocnemius ▶▶

Step into a lunge position, and push the heel of the back leg down into the floor, keeping the back leg straight. Feel the stretch in the upper calf.

sore neck?

The bent-over position of cycling can leave you with a sore neck. To loosen it up, try this routine:

1 Slowly look up to the sky, pushing your chin out.

2 Roll your head down until your chin touches your chest. Place your hands on your head and let their weight stretch the back of the neck.

3 Look forward, then turn and look over your right shoulder as far as possible. Repeat to the left.

4 Look forward, then tilt your head to the right (use the hand on the side of your head to increase the stretch). Repeat to the left.

quadriceps ▸▸

Stand on one leg (steady yourself with one hand on a wall if necessary). Bend the other leg until your heel is close to your butt. Hold your ankle and push your pelvis forward to feel the stretch in the front of the thigh.

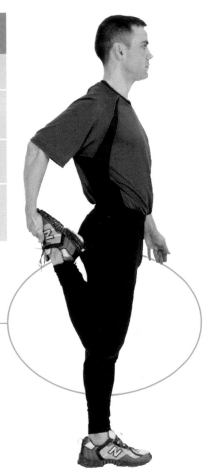

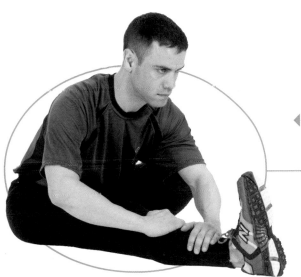

◂◂ hamstrings

Sit on the floor with one leg straight out in front of you and the other bent into the knee of the straight leg. Reach forward toward your toes, keeping your back straight. Feel the stretch above the knee at the back of the straight leg.

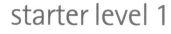

starter level 1

If you're a total beginner, this is where you should start. The most important things for you to do in this first month are to get used to riding and to enjoy your new-found activity. The goal for the next four weeks is to build up to be able to ride for one hour without stopping. At the start, this will seem impossible, but you'll find your endurance improves dramatically in a short space of time. If you're already quite fit, you might be tempted to push harder. Don't—there's no hurry.

Train to your heart rate. See pp. 42–43 for the heart rates and effort levels of the different sessions.

starting out

- Take it easy—aim to finish each session feeling that you could do more.

- But not too easy—ride steady (see p. 42) but don't push yourself.

- Choose quiet roads or country lanes for your riding (see "a sense of place," right).

- Wear a heart rate monitor.

- Spin a small gear quickly instead of pushing a big gear slowly.

- Enjoy it! Cycling is supposed to be fun.

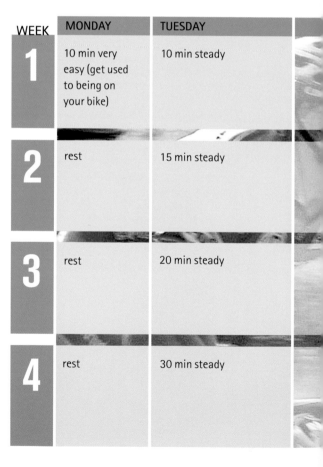

WEEK	MONDAY	TUESDAY
1	10 min very easy (get used to being on your bike)	10 min steady
2	rest	15 min steady
3	rest	20 min steady
4	rest	30 min steady

what if... I'm really strong?

Some people are naturally fitter than others. Everyone has his or her own level and for some, riding at 15 or 20 mph (25 or 30 km/h) is no problem. If you're one of those lucky few, you'll find that this first month is hardly a challenge. You should still do it, though. Overestimating your abilities and pushing too hard are common new-rider mistakes. So keep your effort under control (using a heart rate monitor is a good way to monitor your pace, see p. 23); you don't want to burn yourself out.

a sense of place

One of the most important things to consider when you're training is the route you take. The more bumps, hills, and mountains you have to climb, the harder it will be. Similarly, the more traffic there is, the more intimidating—and dangerous—cycling becomes.

When you're getting started, it's best to find routes that are reasonably flat or, at most, gently undulating (see p. 45 for details of how to describe a route). Anything more and you'll find riding too hard, and might be tempted to give up.

WEDNESDAY	THURSDAY	FRIDAY	SATURDAY	SUNDAY
rest	10 min steady	rest	rest	20 min endurance
rest	25 min steady	rest	15 min steady	30 min endurance
rest	30 min steady	rest	20 min steady	45 min endurance
rest	45 min steady	rest	rest	60 min endurance

2

starter level 2

The two schedules in this level are for riders who can ride for an hour and feel like they "belong" on a bike. These are the schedules you should use after you have successfully completed the level one starter schedule and are eager to go a little farther for a little longer. Don't start your cycling career with these schedules. Total beginners should start with Starter Level I.

doubling up

The program below is designed to work solely on your endurance, bringing you up to a two-hour ride in just four weeks, while the second (over the page) introduces interval training and other achievable "training" rides. You will still be riding four times a week.

tip...

The real trick when building endurance for the first time is to concentrate on endurance alone. So don't be tempted to push yourself beyond the suggested intensity (see pp. 42–43). Concentrate on enjoying the scenery and the freedom that your bike offers.

week 2 – how's it going?

Take a moment at the end of Week 2 to review your progress. How are you coping? If you're feeling unusually tired or sore, you may want to slow your progress by doing each week twice before you move on. Many riders feel that they are not keeping up, and begin to get discouraged. From there it's a short step to putting your bike somewhere out of sight and denying yourself the fitness, freedom, and enjoyment that regular riding can offer. Have a little faith in yourself and keep pedaling away—things will get better.

If you're finding it easy, great, but don't get overconfident and don't start pushing harder just because you think you can. Slow and steady is the key.

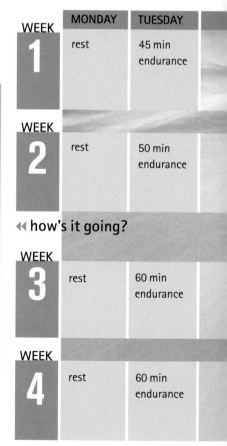

WEEK	MONDAY	TUESDAY	
1	rest	45 min endurance	
2	rest	50 min endurance	

◀◀ **how's it going?**

WEEK			
3	rest	60 min endurance	
4	rest	60 min endurance	

action replay

If you want to stay with this schedule for an extra month or two before you move on, feel free to do so. It's designed to be repeatable, and makes an excellent base fitness program for a new rider to follow over the winter. But if you're going to repeat it, try adding five minutes to each ride. This will further increase your endurance, and will stop your development from leveling off too quickly.

WEDNESDAY	THURSDAY	FRIDAY	SATURDAY	SUNDAY
rest	45 min endurance	rest	15 min warm-up, 20 min steady, 5–15 min cool-down	60 min endurance
rest	50 min endurance	rest	15 min warm-up, 20–30 min steady, 5–15 min cool-down	75 min endurance
rest	60 min endurance	rest	15 min warm-up, 25–30 min steady, 5–15 min cool-down	90 min endurance
rest	15 min warm-up, 30 min steady, 5–15 min cool-down	rest	rest	2 hr endurance

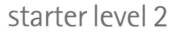

starter level 2

Once you're happy riding for two hours at an endurance-building pace, you can start thinking about adding some faster riding to your program. Faster riding can be done in two ways. It is possible, and sometimes even beneficial, to go hard for an entire ride. But this is something that only fit and experienced riders should attempt. It's better, particularly for new riders, to divide hard work into blocks, separated by periods of recovery, which as we have seen, is called interval training (see p. 43 for more details). This can be very demanding. But it's also the most effective way to get faster and fitter.

what pace?

It can be hard to pace interval training. If you push too hard in the early repetitions you may struggle to finish the later ones. Equally, at the end of the session, you don't want to feel as if you haven't worked hard enough.

- Go by feel on the first effort; your heart rate will lag behind your actual workload.

- Monitor your effort by heart rate, not speed. Headwinds, crosswinds, inclines, and road surfaces will all change the speed you travel for the same amount of effort.

- Start each repetition steadily and increase the pace once you're underway. Go too quickly at the start and you'll soon be exhausted.

- Push hard, but not flat out, in the final stages of your last repetition. Aim to finish the session feeling as if you have worked hard, but could manage one last effort.

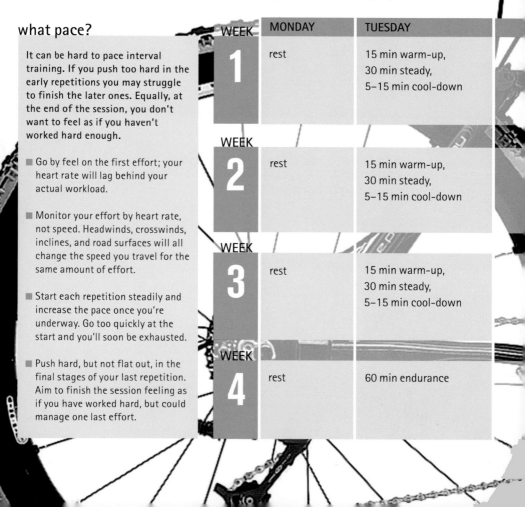

WEEK	MONDAY	TUESDAY
1	rest	15 min warm-up, 30 min steady, 5–15 min cool-down
2	rest	15 min warm-up, 30 min steady, 5–15 min cool-down
3	rest	15 min warm-up, 30 min steady, 5–15 min cool-down
4	rest	60 min endurance

time test

The test at the end of Week 4 will give you an idea of your new abilities. Here's how to do the test:

- Plan a flat route of 5 miles (8 km). Use roads with light traffic and complete your ride in daylight.
- Warm-up by pushing a small gear for 15 to 20 minutes.
- When you reach the start of your course, roll to your start point and begin.
- Gradually build up to a hard but sustainable pace in the first few minutes.

- Try to maintain the same effort all the way, changing gears as necessary.
- Try to lift your pace a little bit further in the final minutes.
- Record your time, speed, and average and maximum heart rates.
- Congratulate yourself on a good hard ride.

Repeat the test every one or two months to see how you are improving. As your fitness and experience improves, you can switch to using a 10-mile (16-km) time trial for your test.

WEDNESDAY	THURSDAY	FRIDAY	SATURDAY	SUNDAY
rest	15 min warm-up, 6 x 1-min speed work with 2-min recoveries, 15 min cool-down	rest	30–45 min recovery	60 min endurance
rest	15 min warm-up, 5 x 2-min speed work with 2-min recoveries, 15 min cool-down	rest	30–45 min recovery	75 min endurance
rest	15 min warm-up, 4 x 3-min speed work with 3-min recoveries, 15 min cool-down	rest	30–45 min recovery	90 min endurance
rest	15 min warm-up, 6 x 1-min speed work with 2-min recoveries, 15 min cool-down	rest	rest	5-mile (8-km) time test

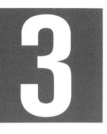

refresher level

By now, you've completed all the starter levels. You're comfortable being on your bike for about an hour several times a week, and even longer on some days. You're looking for a new challenge, but you still feel a little intimidated by the idea of competing at your local cycle club. If you're returning to cycling after a break of more than a couple of months, you can also begin your comeback here.

This four-week schedule is the first in a series of four repeatable programs for general maintenance and winter training. This one is specifically aimed at easing into riding with a club.

These schedules involve regular interval work. Remember to warm up first. Start out at recovery pace, and gradually build up to the effort level required by your main session.

		MONDAY	TUESDAY		WEDNESDAY
WEEK	1	rest	20 min warm-up, 4 x 4-min tempo with 2-min recoveries, 20 min cool-down		rest or 30–45 min recovery
WEEK	2	rest	15 min warm-up, 30–40 min steady, 15 min cool-down		rest or 30–45 min recovery
WEEK	3	rest	20 min warm-up, 3 x 5-min tempo with 2-min recoveries, 20 min cool-down		rest or 30–45 min recovery
WEEK	4	rest	15 min warm-up, 4 x 3-min speed work with 2-min recoveries, 15 min cool-down		rest or 30–45 min recovery

get clubbed, not beaten

It's very important when you start riding with a club that you let them know exactly what your capabilities are. They will probably have a club captain/ride leader, and may even have a coach you can talk to. Phone in advance of going along to a ride to get the low down. A good club will have groups organized by speed. Just slot into the right one and start making friends. And in the unlikely event that you do get dropped off the back of the group, don't be disheartened. Keep on training and you will be able to keep up.

repeating the program

To add an extra challenge to this schedule, repeat the whole four-week block, adding 10 minutes to each steady or endurance ride, and an extra repetition to each tempo and speed work ride.

THURSDAY	FRIDAY	SATURDAY	SUNDAY
60 min endurance	rest	15 min warm-up, 30 min steady, 15 min cool-down	1 hr 30 min to 2 hr endurance
60–75 min endurance	rest	15 min warm-up, 30 min steady, 15 min cool-down	1 hr 45 min to 2 hr 30 min endurance
75 min endurance	rest	15 min warm-up, 30 min steady, 15 min cool-down	2 hr to 2 hr 45 min endurance or first long ride with club (take it easy)
60 min endurance, including 4 x 15-sec sprints with 5-min recoveries	rest	30–45 min recovery	2 hr 30 min endurance or long ride with club (take it easy)

3

refresher level

The second refresher level schedule challenges you with your first longer-term goal. Over 10 weeks, it takes you from your current endurance level to a sub-six hour, 100-mile (160-km) ride. That may sound

WEEK	MONDAY	TUESDAY	
1	rest or 30 min recovery	15 min warm-up, 30 min steady, 15 min cool-down	
2	rest	15 min warm-up, 35 min steady, 15 min cool-down	
3	rest	15 min warm-up, 40 min steady, 15 min cool-down	
4	rest	15 min warm-up, 30 min steady, 15 min cool-down	
5	rest	15 min warm-up, 45 min steady, 15 min cool-down	
6	rest	15 min warm-up, 45 min steady, 15 min cool-down	
7	rest	15 min warm-up, 50 min steady, 15 min cool-down	
8	rest	15 min warm-up, 40 min steady, 15 min cool-down	
9	rest	15 min warm-up, 50 min steady, 15 min cool-down	
10	rest	15 min warm-up, 30 min steady, 15 min cool-down	

As we have seen, a century is simply a 100-mile (160-km) ride. It could be an informal session with friends, an event put on by a touring club, or a road race. There are even 100-mile (160-km) time trials.

impossible, but have faith—it's surprising how well you can build up to long-distance riding. The program also works well as a late winter endurance booster.

pace

■ Your endurance pace should be your target century pace. This may mean pushing a little harder on Sundays than you have been, but don't push too hard.
■ Your steady sessions will build gradually. Always ride at the same intensity (see p. 42).

WEDNESDAY	THURSDAY	FRIDAY	SATURDAY	SUNDAY
rest or 30–45 min recovery	15 min warm-up, 30 min steady, 15 min cool-down	rest	1 hr endurance	45 miles (70 km) endurance
rest or 30–45 min recovery	15 min warm-up, 35 min steady, 15 min cool-down	rest	1 hr 5 min endurance	50 miles (80 km) endurance
rest or 30–45 min recovery	15 min warm-up, 40 min steady, 15 min cool-down	rest	1 hr 10 min endurance	55 miles (90 km) endurance
rest or 30–45 min recovery	15 min warm-up, 4 x 4-min tempo with 2-min recoveries, 15 min cool-down	rest	1 hr endurance	50 miles (80 km) endurance
rest or 30–45 min recovery	15 min warm-up, 45 min steady, 15 min cool-down	rest	1 hr 10 min endurance	60 miles (95 km) endurance
rest or 30–45 min recovery	15 min warm-up, 45 min steady, 15 min cool-down	rest	1 hr 15 min endurance	65 miles (100 km) endurance
rest or 30–45 min recovery	15 min warm-up, 50 min steady, 15 min cool-down	rest	1 hr 20 min endurance	70 miles (110 km) endurance
rest or 30–45 min recovery	15 min warm-up, 3 x 5-min tempo with 2-min recoveries, 15 min cool-down	rest	1 hr 10 min endurance	60 miles (95 km) endurance
rest or 30 min recovery	15 min warm-up, 50 min steady, 15 min cool-down	rest	1 hr 15 min endurance	75 miles (120 km) endurance
rest or 30 min recovery	15 min warm-up, 30 min steady, 15 min cool-down	rest	20–30 min recovery	Century (100 miles/ 160 km)

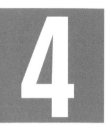

intermediate level

By the time you reach this level, you should be used to spending long periods in the saddle and training four to six times per week for more than two hours at a time. You should be capable of good bursts of speed, enough to keep your clubmates on their guard. You should feel confident and strong and ready to start proving yourself in races. The three schedules in this level cover: (a) basic, repeatable training that allows you to pick and choose races at your leisure; (b) riding a century for a time target of your choice; and (c) an introduction to the high-speed world of time trials.

You may be training with friends or clubmates several times a week. But don't push yourself beyond your capabilities. By all means tailor your training to fit in with club rides and so on, but still follow every hard ride with a rest or recovery day. Know your heart rate zones and work to them, not to the pace of others.

WEEK	MONDAY	TUESDAY
1	rest	15 min warm-up, 3 x 8-min tempo with 2-min recoveries, or 6 x 3-min hill strength with 2-min recoveries, 15 min cool-down
2	rest	15 min warm-up, 45-60 min steady, 15 min cool-down
3	rest	15 min warm-up, 3 x 8-min tempo with 2-min recoveries, or 6 x 3-min hill strength with 2-min recoveries, 15 min cool-down
4	rest	15 min warm-up, 4 x 3-min speed work with 2-min recoveries, 15 min cool-down

train to the beat

Train to your heart rate (see pp. 42–43). Your pace will gradually improve as you get fitter, but your heart rate should stay the same. To add an extra challenge to this schedule, repeat the four-week block, adding 10-15 minutes to each steady or endurance ride, and an extra repetition to each tempo and speed work ride.

WEDNESDAY	THURSDAY	FRIDAY	SATURDAY	SUNDAY
rest or 30-45 min recovery	60-90 min endurance	rest or 30-45 min recovery	15 min warm-up, 40 min steady, 15 min cool-down	2 hr to 2 hr 30 min endurance
rest or 30-45 min recovery	60-90 min endurance	rest or 30-45 min recovery	15 min warm-up, 40 min steady, 15 min cool-down	2 hr to 2 hr 45 min endurance
rest or 30-45 min recovery	75 min endurance	rest or 30-45 min recovery	15 min warm-up, 40 min steady, 15 min cool-down	2 hr to 3 hr endurance
rest or 30-45 min recovery	60 min endurance, include 5 x 15-sec sprints with 4-min recoveries	rest or 30-45 min recovery	30-45 min recovery	2 hr 30 min endurance or race

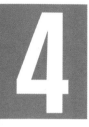

racing the century: 100 miles (160 km)

You will be covering a high mileage during this schedule, so be prepared to feel tired. Train carefully and always take the rest option on easy days if you feel fatigued or your legs feel sore.

week 4— how's it going?

Are you feeling strong? If you want a greater challenge, add an extra 15–30 minutes to each steady Saturday ride.

⏶ **how's it going?**

WEEK	MONDAY	TUESDAY	WEDNESDAY
1	rest	15 min warm-up, 4 x 6-min tempo with 2-min recoveries, 15 min cool-down	rest or 30–45 min recovery
2	rest	15 min warm-up, 4 x 6-min tempo with 2-min recoveries, 15 min cool-down	rest or 30–45 min recovery
3	rest	15 min warm-up, 3 x 8-min tempo with 2-min recoveries, 15 min cool-down	rest or 30–45 min recovery
4	rest	15 min warm-up, 5 x 3-min speed work with 2-min recoveries, 15 min cool-down	rest or 30–45 min recovery
5	rest	15 min warm-up, 3 x 8-min tempo with 2-min recoveries, 15 min cool-down	rest or 30–45 min recovery
6	rest	15 min warm-up, 2 x 9-min tempo with 5-min recoveries, 15 min cool-down	rest or 30–45 min recovery
7	rest	15 min warm-up, 2 x 10-min tempo with 5-min recoveries, 15 min cool-down	rest or 30–45 min recovery
8	rest	15 min warm-up, 5 x 3-min speed work with 2-min recoveries, 15 min cool-down	rest or 30–45 min recovery
9	rest	15 min warm-up, 3 x 8-min tempo with 2-min recoveries, 15 min cool-down	rest or 30–45 min recovery
10	rest	15 min warm-up, 3 x 8-min tempo with 2-min recoveries, 15 min cool-down	rest

THURSDAY	FRIDAY	SATURDAY	SUNDAY
60-90 min endurance	rest or 30-45 min recovery	15 min warm-up, 40 min steady, 15 min cool-down	50 miles (80 km) endurance
60-90 min endurance	rest or 30-45 min recovery	15 min warm-up, 45 min steady, 15 min cool-down	55 miles (90 km) endurance
60-90 min endurance	rest or 30-45 min recovery	15 min warm-up, 50 min steady, 15 min cool-down	60 miles (100 km) endurance
60 min endurance	rest or 30-45 min recovery	15 min warm-up, 30 min steady, 15 min cool-down	55 miles (90 km) endurance
75-120 min endurance	rest or 30-45 min recovery	15 min warm-up, 45 min steady, 15 min cool-down	65 miles (105 km) endurance
75-120 min endurance	rest or 30-45 min recovery	15 min warm-up, 50 min steady, 15 min cool-down	70 miles (110 km) endurance
75-120 min endurance	rest or 30-45 min recovery	15 min warm-up, 50 min steady, 15 min cool-down	75 miles (120 km) endurance
60 min endurance	rest or 30-45 min recovery	15 min warm-up, 60 min steady, 15 min cool-down	80 miles (130 km) endurance
60-90 min endurance	rest or 30-45 min recovery	15 min warm-up, 40 min steady, 15 min cool-down	70 miles (110 km) endurance
15 min warm-up, 30 min steady, 15 min cool-down	rest	30-45 min recovery	Century (160 km)

week 8 – how's it going?

By now you should have a reasonable grasp of your century capabilities. If everything is going well and you feel strong, aim to race your century at your steady training pace. If you're struggling to complete your long rides at this pace, consider riding at your endurance pace instead.

⏶ how's it going?

4

10-mile (16-km) time trial

With all their flashy kit and single-minded reputation, time trialists can seem intimidating. Do not be deceived—they were all novices once.

WEEK	MONDAY	TUESDAY		WEDNESDAY
1	rest	15 min warm-up, 6 x 3-min flat strength with 2-min spin recoveries, 15 min cool-down		rest or 30-45 min recovery
2	rest	15 min warm-up, 6 x 3-min flat strength with 2-min spin recoveries, 15 min cool-down		rest or 30-45 min recovery
3	rest	15 min warm-up, 5 x 4-min flat strength with 2-min spin recoveries, 15 min cool-down		rest or 30-45 min recovery
4	rest	15 min warm-up, 6 x 3-min flat strength with 2-min spin recoveries, 15 min cool-down		rest or 30-45 min recovery

◀◀ how's it going?

5	rest	15 min warm-up, 3 x 8-min tempo with 2-min recoveries, 15 min cool-down		rest or 30-45 min recovery
6	rest	15 min warm-up, 2 x 10-min tempo with 10-min recovery, 15 min cool-down		rest or 30-45 min recovery
7	rest	15 min warm-up, 2 x 12-min tempo with 5-min recovery, 15 min cool-down		rest or 30-45 min recovery
8	rest	15 min warm-up, 2 x 15-min tempo with 5-min recovery, 15 min cool-down		rest or 30-45 min recovery
9	rest	15 min warm-up, 2 x 10-min tempo with 10-min recovery, 15 min cool-down		rest or 30-45 min recovery
10	rest	15 min warm-up, 2 x 2 miles (3.2 km) at target race pace with a 10-min recovery, 15 min cool-down		rest

week 4 – how's it going?

How's it going? If you want to test your pace, do a 10-mile (16-km) test (see pp. 40-41) instead of your steady Saturday ride, then ride two hours recovery on Sunday. Remember to warm-up fully beforehand (see below).

30+ minutes
Don't worry it's early days yet.
30-28 minutes
Good work so far, keep it up.
28-25 minutes
A strong performance already.
25 or less
You're flying! You must have a talent for this. But don't push too hard too soon.

the warm-up

A proper warm-up is essential if you want to reach your potential. Here are five tips for a good warm-up:

- Never rush a warm-up. Try to spend 30 to 60 minutes on it.
- Keep hydrated during your warm-up. Sip a drink every five minutes.
- Spin a small gear to start. Spend about 15 minutes loosening your muscles.
- Lift your heart rate to the level you want to race at, but only for short bursts (30 to 90 seconds) and with long recoveries.
- End your warm-up at the start point, but also leave a few minutes for pre-race relaxation.

THURSDAY	FRIDAY	SATURDAY	SUNDAY
15 min warm-up, 3 x 1 mile (1.6 km) at target race pace with 5-min recoveries, 15 min cool-down	rest or 30-45 min recovery	15 min warm-up, 40 min steady, 15 min cool-down	2 hr to 2 hr 30 min endurance
15 min warm-up, 2 x 2 miles (3.2 km) at target race pace with a 10-min recovery, 15 min cool-down	rest or 30-45 min recovery	15 min warm-up, 40 min steady, 15 min cool-down	2 hr to 2 hr 30 min endurance
15 min warm-up, 2 x 3 miles (5 km) at target race pace with a 10-min recovery, 15 min cool-down	rest or 30-45 min recovery	15 min warm-up, 40 min steady, 15 min cool-down	2 hr to 2 hr 30 min endurance
15 min warm-up, one each of 3 miles (5 km), 2 miles (3.2 km), and 1 mile (1.6 km) at target race pace with a 10-min recovery, 15 min cool-down	rest or 30-45 min recovery	15 min warm-up, 30 min steady, 15 min cool-down	2 hr endurance
15 min warm-up, 2 x 4 miles (6.5 km) at target race pace with a 10-min recovery, 15 min cool-down	rest or 30-45 min recovery	15 min warm-up, 40 min steady, 15 min cool-down	2 hr to 2 hr 30 min endurance
15 min warm-up, 2 x 4 miles (6.5 km) at target race pace with a 5-min recovery, 15 min cool-down	rest or 30-45 min recovery	15 min warm-up, 40 min steady, 15 min cool-down	2 hr to 2 hr 30 min endurance
15 min warm-up, 2 x 4 miles (6.5 km) at target race pace with a 5-min recovery, 15 min cool-down	rest or 30-45 min recovery	15 min warm-up, 40 min steady, 15 min cool-down	2 hr to 2 hr 30 min endurance
15 min warm-up, 2 x 4 miles (6.5 km) at target race pace with a 5-min recovery, 15 min cool-down	rest or 30-45 min recovery	15 min warm-up, 30 min steady, 15 min cool-down	2 hr to 2 hr 30 min endurance
15 min warm-up, 6 miles (10 km) at target race pace, 15 min cool-down	rest or 30-45 min recovery	15 min warm-up, 40 min steady, 15 min cool-down	2 hr endurance
15 min warm-up, 40 min steady, 15 min cool-down	rest	30-45 min recovery	10-mile (16-km) time trial

5 expert level 1

The three schedules at this level are designed for riders with a season of racing experience. You should now have done the base building, added some speed, and tried your hand at a few local time trials and club races. But you can still improve. Again, there's a repeatable schedule you can use to

WEEK				
1	rest	15 min warm-up, 45 min steady, 15 min cool-down	rest or 1–2 hr recovery	
2	rest	15 min warm-up, 3 x 10-min tempo with 5-min recoveries, 15 min cool-down	rest or 1–2 hr recovery	
3	rest	15 min warm-up, 3 x 10-min tempo with 5-min recoveries, 15 min cool-down	rest or 1–2 hr recovery	
4	rest	15 min warm-up, 4 x 3-min speed work with 2-min recoveries, 15 min cool-down	rest or 1–2 hr recovery	

tip...

If you want to race on Sunday of week four, take Friday as a total rest day and do 30 minutes recovery riding in a small gear to loosen your legs on Saturday.

build fitness over the winter, and if you want to race casually, there are also specific 10-week schedules designed to prepare you for two specific goals—your first attempt at a 25-mile (40-km) time trial, and at a criterium.

added challenge

As for the basic intermediate schedule, add an extra challenge to this schedule by repeating the four-week block, adding 15–20 minutes to each steady or endurance ride, and an extra repetition to each tempo and speed work ride.

1 hr to 1 hr 30 min hilly endurance ride	rest or 1 hr recovery	15 min warm-up, 45 min steady, 15 min cool-down	2 hr 30 min endurance
1 hr to 1 hr 30 min hilly endurance ride	rest or 1 hr recovery	15 min warm-up, 45–60 min steady, 15 min cool-down	2 hr 45 min endurance
1 hr to 1 hr 30 min hilly endurance ride	rest or 1 hr recovery	15 min warm-up, 60 min steady, 15 min cool-down	3 hr endurance
1–2 hr endurance, include 2 sets of 3 x 15 sec sprints (some on hills) with 2-min recoveries (10–20 min between sets)	rest or 1 hr recovery	rest or 30–90 min recovery	3 hr 15 min endurance or race

5

the trial: 25-mile (40-km) time trial

The 25-mile (40-km) time trial is a race aimed squarely at the purist. It is short enough to race flat out, but long enough to reward the careful rider.

week 8— how's it going?

How did you perform in the 10-mile (16-km) time trial, known in racing slang as the "10" (or the "25" for the 25-mile (40-km) distance)? Hopefully, you rode at least at your target 25-mile (40-km) pace. If you were more than a minute off that pace, consider setting a slightly easier target. If you rode at a 25-mile (40-km) pace the whole way, did you find it easy? Could you maintain that pace for more than double the distance? Set your targets according to how you performed.

WEEK	MONDAY	TUESDAY	WEDNESDAY	
1	rest	15 min warm-up, 3 x 8-min flat strength with 2-min spin recoveries, 15 min cool-down	rest or 1–2 hr recovery	
2	rest	15 min warm-up, 3 x 8-min flat strength with 2-min spin recoveries, 15 min cool-down	rest or 1–2 hr recovery	
3	rest	15 min warm-up, 3 x 8-min flat strength with 2-min spin recoveries, 15 min cool-down	rest or 1–2 hr recovery	
4	rest	15 min warm-up, 5 x 3-min speed work with 3-min recoveries, 15 min cool-down	rest or 1 hr recovery	
5	rest	15 min warm-up, 5 x 4-min speed work with 2-min recoveries, 15 min cool-down	rest or 1–2 hr recovery	
6	rest	15 min warm-up, 5 x 4-min speed work with 2-min recoveries, 15 min cool-down	rest or 1–2 hr recovery	
7	rest	15 min warm-up, 4 x 5-min speed work with 3-min recoveries, 15 min cool-down	rest or 1–2 hr recovery	
8	rest	15 min warm-up, 4 x 5-min speed work with 3-min recoveries, 15 min cool-down	rest or 1–2 hr recovery	

⌃ how's it going?

WEEK	MONDAY	TUESDAY	WEDNESDAY	
9	rest	15 min warm-up, 5 x 3 min speed work with 3-min recoveries, 15 min cool-down	rest or 1–2 hr recovery	
10	rest	15 min warm-up, 5 x 3 min speed work with 3-min recoveries, 15 min cool-down	rest	

One hour or less of pure, uninterrupted effort. Some people find it boring, others love the focus the race demands. The only way to tell is to try one.

Do all your quality training sessions and your Saturday rides on your own and in your time-trial position (see pp. 52–53).

THURSDAY	FRIDAY	SATURDAY	SUNDAY
15 min warm-up, 2 x 3 miles (5 km) at target race pace with 5-min recoveries, 15 min cool-down	rest or 30–45 min recovery	15 min warm-up, 1 hr hilly steady, 15 min cool-down	2 hr 30 min to 3 hr endurance
15 min warm-up, 2 x 4 miles (6.5 km) at target race pace with 5-min recovery, 15 min cool-down	rest or 30–45 min recovery	15 min warm-up, 1 hr hilly steady, 15 min cool-down	2 hr 45 min to 3 hr endurance
15 min warm-up, 2 x 5 miles (8 km) at target race pace with 5-min recovery, 15 min cool-down	rest or 30–45 min recovery	15 min warm-up, 1 hr hilly steady, 15 min cool-down	3 hr endurance
15 min warm-up, 1 hr hilly steady, 15 min cool-down	rest or 1 hr recovery	rest or 30–45 min recovery	10-mile (16-km) time trial
15 min warm-up, 2 x 6 miles (10 km) at target race pace with a 5-min recovery, 15 min cool-down	rest or 30–45 min recovery	15 min warm-up, 3 x 10-min tempo with 5-min recoveries, 15 min cool-down	3 hr endurance
15 min warm-up, 2 x 8 miles (13 km) at target race pace with a 5-min recovery, 15 min cool-down	rest or 30–45 min recovery	15 min warm-up, 3 x 10-min tempo with 5-min recoveries, 15 min cool-down	3 hr endurance
15 min warm-up, 2 x 8 miles (13 km) at target race pace with a 5-min recovery, 15 min cool-down	rest or 30–45 min recovery	15 min warm-up, 3 x 10-min tempo with 5-min recoveries, 15 min cool-down	3 hr endurance
15 min warm-up, 2 x 4 miles (6.5 km) at target race pace with a 5-min recovery, 15 min cool-down	rest or 1 hr recovery	rest or 30–45 min recovery	10-mile (16-km) time trial
15 min warm-up, 2 x 6 miles (10 km) at target race pace with a 10-min recovery, 15 min cool-down	rest or 1 hr recovery	rest or 30–45 min recovery	10-mile (16-km) time trial (at target 25-mile (40-km) pace)
15 min warm-up, 2 x 4 miles (6.5 km) at target race pace with a 10-min recovery, 15 min cool-down	rest	30–45 min recovery	

5

criterium racing

Criteriums are comparatively short, fast, multilap races that involve lots of technical cornering and climbs. The pace will vary a lot during the race.

tip...

Try to train on a course similar to your goal race. Include plenty of training with other riders, and practice taking corners and short hills at speed.

WEEK				
1	rest	15 min warm-up, 4 x 15-min build pace endurance to hard, 15 min cool-down	rest or 1–2 hr recovery	
2	rest	15 min warm-up, 4 x 15-min build pace endurance to hard, 15 min cool-down	rest or 1–2 hr recovery	
3	rest	15 min warm-up, 3 x 20-min build pace endurance to hard, 15 min cool-down	rest or 1–2 hr recovery	
4	rest	15 min warm-up, 5 x 4-min speed work with 1-min recoveries, 15 min cool-down	rest or 1–2 hr recovery	

week 4— how's it going?

This program contains lots of high-intensity speed work and sprints. If your legs feel heavy or you feel unusually tired, reduce the amount of riding you do on your recovery days or even take days of complete rest. Make sure you stretch and consider getting regular massage to help you relax.

◀◀ how's it going?

WEEK				
5	rest	15 min warm-up, 3 x 20-min build pace endurance to hard, 15 min cool-down	rest or 1–2 hr recovery	
6	rest	20 min warm-up, 2 x 25-min build pace endurance to hard, 20 min cool-down	rest or 1–2 hr recovery	
7	rest	15 min warm-up, 2 x 30-min build pace endurance to hard, 15 min cool-down	rest or 1–2 hr recovery	
8	rest	15 min warm-up, 2 x 30-min build pace endurance to hard, 15 min cool-down	rest or 1–2 hr recovery	
9	rest	15 min warm-up, 6 x 3-min speed work with 2-min recoveries, 15 min cool-down	rest or 1–2 hr recovery	
10	rest	15 min warm-up, 1 hr steady including 10 x 10-sec sprints with 2-min recoveries, 15 min cool-down	rest	

One moment you'll be cruising at
18 mph (30 km/h), the next someone
will attack at the front and the pace
will leap to well over 25 mph (40 km/h).

15 min warm-up, 1 hr steady including 6 x 15-sec sprints with 5-min recoveries, 15 min cool-down	rest or 1 hr recovery	15 min warm-up, 1 hr hilly steady, 15 min cool-down	2 hr 30 min to 3 hr endurance
15 min warm-up, 1 hr steady including 6 x 10–20-sec uphill sprints with 5-min recoveries, 15 min cool-down	rest or 1 hr recovery	15 min warm-up, 1 hr hilly steady, 15 min cool-down	2 hr 45 min to 3 hr endurance
15 min warm-up, 1 hr steady including 10 x 10-sec sprints with 2-min recoveries, 15 min cool-down	rest or 1 hr recovery	15 min warm-up, 1 hr hilly steady, 15 min cool-down	3 hr endurance
15 min warm-up, 1 hr steady including 6 x 20–30-sec sprints in a low gear with 5 to 10-min recoveries, 15 min cool-down	rest or 1 hr recovery	rest or 30–45 min recovery	2 hr 30 min endurance or 10-mile (16-km) time trial (on normal race bike)
15 min warm-up, 1 hr steady including 2 sets of 5 x 15-sec sprints with 2-min recoveries (leave 10–15 min between sets), 15 min cool-down	rest or 1 hr recovery	30 min warm-up, 30 min group tempo, 30 min cool-down	3 hr endurance
15 min warm-up, 1 hr steady including 6 x 15–20-sec sprints with 2-min recoveries (alternate your biggest and smallest gear), 15 min cool-down	rest or 1 hr recovery	30 min warm-up, 35 min group tempo, 30 min cool-down	3 hr endurance
15 min warm-up, 1 hr steady including 2 sets of 5 x 10-sec sprints (from close to a stop) with 2-min recoveries (take 10–15 min between sets), 15 min cool-down	rest or 1 hr recovery	30 min warm-up, 40 min group tempo, 30 min cool-down	3 hr endurance
15 min warm-up, 1 hr steady including 6 x 20–40-sec sprints off the bottom of a hill, 15 min cool-down	rest or 1 hr recovery	rest or 30–45 min recovery	10-mile (16-km) time trial (on normal race bike)
15 min warm-up, 1 hr steady including 10 x 10-sec sprints with 2-min recoveries, 15 min cool-down	rest or 1 hr recovery	15 min warm-up, 30 min tempo, 15 min cool-down	3 hr endurance
15 min warm-up, 30 min steady, 15 min cool-down	rest	30–45 min recovery	

6

expert level 2

Once you've reached a level where you're racing frequently, it's tempting to think that you know it all. You don't. There's always room for improvement. Up to now, all the schedules (other than the repeatable four-week ones) have focused on reaching a single goal. It's a great way to improve, but perhaps not the best way to improve as a racer. Simply put, there are too many chances in a race for things to go wrong. You may have a bad

train to your weaknesses

If you're a sprinter and flat road rider, focus your sessions on smaller gears, hillier routes, and climbing speed work. If you fly up hills but struggle in a sprint, swap your speed work for sprints with short recoveries.

added challenge

As for the previous intermediate and expert level, add an extra challenge to this schedule by repeating the four-week block, adding 15–30 minutes to each steady or endurance ride, and an extra repetition to each tempo and speed work ride.

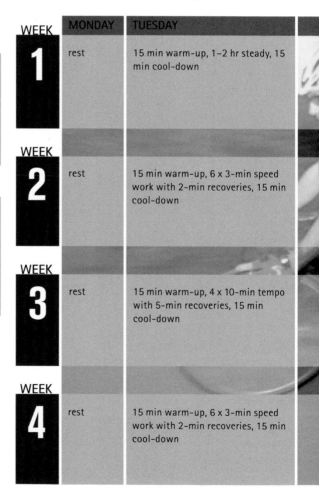

WEEK	MONDAY	TUESDAY
1	rest	15 min warm-up, 1–2 hr steady, 15 min cool-down
2	rest	15 min warm-up, 6 x 3-min speed work with 2-min recoveries, 15 min cool-down
3	rest	15 min warm-up, 4 x 10-min tempo with 5-min recoveries, 15 min cool-down
4	rest	15 min warm-up, 6 x 3-min speed work with 2-min recoveries, 15 min cool-down

day, you may miss the break when it goes, you might puncture or even crash.

To race successfully, you need to race frequently, which is where these final schedules will help. Focusing either on time trials or road racing, the two ten-week programs here are designed for an experienced athlete during the racing season. Each is targeted at a final peak performance, with smaller race targets along the way. The programs should only be attempted if you have an endurance base of rides over three hours (probably built over winter and spring) and a season's racing experience.

WEDNESDAY	THURSDAY	FRIDAY	SATURDAY	SUNDAY
rest or 1–3 hr recovery	2–3 hr hilly endurance	rest or 1–2 hr recovery	15 min warm-up, 60 min steady, 15 min cool-down	3 hr endurance
rest or 1–3 hr recovery	2 hr hilly endurance	rest or 1–2 hr recovery	15 min warm-up, 60–75 min steady, 15 min cool-down	3 hr 30 min endurance
rest or 1–3 hr recovery	2–3 hr hilly endurance	rest or 1–2 hr recovery	15 min warm-up, 60–90 min steady, 15 min cool-down	4 hr endurance
rest or 1 hr recovery	2 hr endurance including 2 sets of 4 x 15-sec sprints (some on hills) with 2-min recoveries, 15 min between sets	rest or 1 hr recovery	rest or 30–60 min recovery	4 hr endurance or race

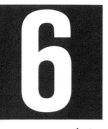

mastering the time trial

◀◀ how's it going?

WEEK	MONDAY	TUESDAY	WEDNESDAY	
1	rest	15 min warm-up, 4 x 10-min tempo with 5-min recoveries, 15 min cool-down	rest or 1–3 hr recovery	
2	rest	30 min warm-up, 6 x 3-min speed work with 2-min recoveries, 30 min cool-down	rest or 1–3 hr recovery	
3	rest	30 min warm-up, 5 x 4-min speed work with 2-min recoveries, 30 min cool-down	rest or 1–3 hr recovery	
4	rest	15 min warm-up, 4 x 10-min tempo with 5-min recoveries, 15 min cool-down	rest or 1–3 hr recovery	
5	rest	30 min warm-up, 6 x 4-min speed work with 1-min recoveries, 30 min cool-down	rest or 1–3 hr recovery	
6	rest	30 min warm-up, 5 x 5-min speed work with 1-min recoveries, 30 min cool-down	rest or 1–3 hr recovery	
7	rest	30 min warm-up, 5 x 5-min speed work with 1-min recoveries, 30 min cool-down	rest or 1–3 hr recovery	
8	rest	30 min warm-up, 4 x 6-min speed work with 2-min recoveries, 30 min cool-down	rest or 1–3 hr recovery	
9	rest	15 min warm-up, 5 x 3-min speed work with 3-min recoveries, 15 min cool-down	rest or 1–2 hr recovery	
10	rest	15 min warm-up, 5 x 3-min speed work with 3-min recoveries, 15 min cool-down	rest	

how's it going?

week 4— how's it going?

Are you breaking the hour for a "25," and 24 minutes for a "10?" If so, it's probably worth trying to buy some extra speed. An individually fitted, time-trial-specific bike with aerodynamic wheels can save you about 30 seconds over 10 miles (16 km). Start saving, though, they are expensive.

tip...

The demands of this much riding are high. Don't train using big gears, and follow the shorter sessions on recovery days. Only race once a week, even though races are listed here all weekend.

THURSDAY	FRIDAY	SATURDAY	SUNDAY
15 min warm-up, 2 x 5 miles (8 km) at target race pace with 5-min recovery, 15 min cool-down	rest or 1 hr recovery	15 min warm-up, 1–2 hr steady, 15 min cool-down	3–4 hr endurance
15 min warm-up, 2 x 6 miles (10 km) at target race pace with 5-min recovery, 15 min cool-down	rest or 1 hr recovery	rest or 1 hr recovery	10-mile (16-km) time trial
15 min warm-up, 2 x 7 miles (11 km) at target 25 pace with 5-min recovery, 15 min cool-down	rest or 1 hr recovery	15 min warm-up, 1–2 hr steady, 15 min cool-down	3–4 hr endurance
15 min warm-up, 10 x 1-min speed work with 2-min recoveries, 15 min cool-down	rest or 1 hr recovery	rest or 1 hr recovery	25-mile (40-km) time trial
15 min warm-up, 2 x 8 miles (13 km) at target 25 pace with a 5-min recovery, 15 min cool-down	rest or 1 hr recovery	15 min warm-up, 1–2 hr steady, 15 min cool-down	3–4 hr endurance
15 min warm-up, 2 x 9 miles (14.5 km) at target 25 pace with a 5-min recovery, 15 min cool-down	rest or 1 hr recovery	30 min warm-up, 35 min group tempo, 30 min cool-down	25-mile (40-km) time trial
15 min warm-up, 2 x 10 miles (16 km) at target 25 pace with a 5-min recovery, 15 min cool-down	rest or 1 hr recovery	15 min warm-up, 1–2 hr steady, 15 min cool-down	3–4 hr endurance
15 min warm-up, 1–2 hr steady, 15 min cool-down	rest or 1 hr recovery	rest or 1 hr recovery	10-mile (16-km) time trial
15 min warm-up, 2 x 8 miles (13 km) at target 25 pace with a 5-min recovery, 15 min cool-down	rest or 1 hr recovery	rest or 1 hr recovery	10-mile (16-km) time trial
15 min warm-up, 3 x 5 miles (8 km) at target 25 pace with 5-min recoveries, 15 min cool-down	rest	30–45 min recovery	**25-mile (40-km) time trial**

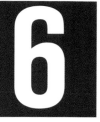

hit the road performances on the road

▼ how's it going?

WEEK	MONDAY	TUESDAY	WEDNESDAY
1	rest	2 hr endurance including 2 sets of 4 x 15-sec sprints (some on hills) with 2-min recoveries, 15 min between sets	rest or 1–3 hr recovery
2	rest	30 min warm-up, 5 x 4-min speed work with 2-min recoveries, 30 min cool-down	rest or 1–3 hr recovery
3	rest	30 min warm-up, 45 min group tempo, 30 min cool-down	rest or 1–3 hr recovery
4	rest	30 min warm-up, 5 x 4-min speed work with 2-min recoveries, 30 min cool-down	rest or 1–3 hr recovery
5	rest	30 min warm-up, 45 min group tempo, 30 min cool-down	rest or 1–3 hr recovery
6	rest	30 min warm-up, 2 x 20-min build pace endurance to hard, 30 min cool-down	rest or 1–3 hr recovery
7	rest	30 min warm-up, 45 min group tempo, 30 min cool-down	rest or 1–3 hr recovery
8	rest	30 min warm-up, 2 x 30-min build pace endurance to hard, 30 min cool-down	rest or 1–3 hr recovery
9	rest	30 min warm-up, 45 min group tempo, 30 min cool-down	rest or 1–2 hr recovery
10	rest	2 hr endurance including 10 x 15-sec sprints with 3-min recoveries	rest

tip...

If you train in a group for speed work and sprints, take turns leading the sprints. The leader starts to sprint without warning and everyone else must follow and try to catch his wheel.

**week 4—
how's it going?**

If you want to race well, you need to race smart. Get to know who the quick riders at your races are. Watch them to see when they make their moves. Then follow—if you can.

THURSDAY	FRIDAY	SATURDAY	SUNDAY
30 min warm-up, 5 x 4-min speed work with 2-min recoveries, 30 min cool-down	rest or 1 hr recovery	15 min warm-up, 1 hr hilly steady, 15 min cool-down	3–4 hr endurance
2 hr endurance including 2 sets of 4 x 15-sec sprints (start each when rounding a corner) with 2-min recoveries, 15 min between sets	rest or 1 hr recovery	rest or 1 hr recovery	10-mile (16-km) time trial
30 min warm-up, 5 x 4-min speed work with 2-min recoveries, 30 min cool-down	rest or 1 hr recovery	15 min warm-up, 1 hr hilly steady, 15 min cool-down	3–4 hr endurance
2 hr endurance including 2 sets of 4 x 15-sec sprints (some on hills) with 2-min recoveries, 15 min between sets	rest or 1 hr recovery	rest or 1 hr recovery	criterium
30 min warm-up, 6 x 4-min speed work with 1-min recoveries, 30 min cool-down	rest or 1 hr recovery	15 min warm-up, 1 hr hilly steady, 15 min cool-down	3–4 hr endurance
30 min warm-up, 1 hr steady including 8 x 15–20-sec sprints with 2-min recoveries (alternate your biggest and smallest gear), 30 min cool-down	rest or 1 hr recovery	rest or 1 hr recovery	criterium
30 min warm-up, 1 hr steady including 2 sets of 5 x 15-sec sprints with 2-min recoveries (roll almost to a stop before each sprint and take 10–15 min between sets), 30 min cool-down	rest or 1 hr recovery	15 min warm-up, 1 hr hilly steady, 15 min cool-down	3–4 hr endurance
30 min warm-up, 1 hr steady including 2 sets of 4 x 15-sec sprints (some on hills) with 2-min recoveries (15 min between sets), 30 min cool-down	rest or 1 hr recovery	rest or 1 hr recovery	criterium
30 min warm-up, 5 x 4-min speed work with 2-min recoveries, 30 min cool-down	rest or 1 hr recovery	rest or 1 hr recovery	10-mile (16-km) time trial (on normal race bike)
15 min warm-up, 45 min group tempo, 15 min cool-down	rest	30–60 min recovery	road race

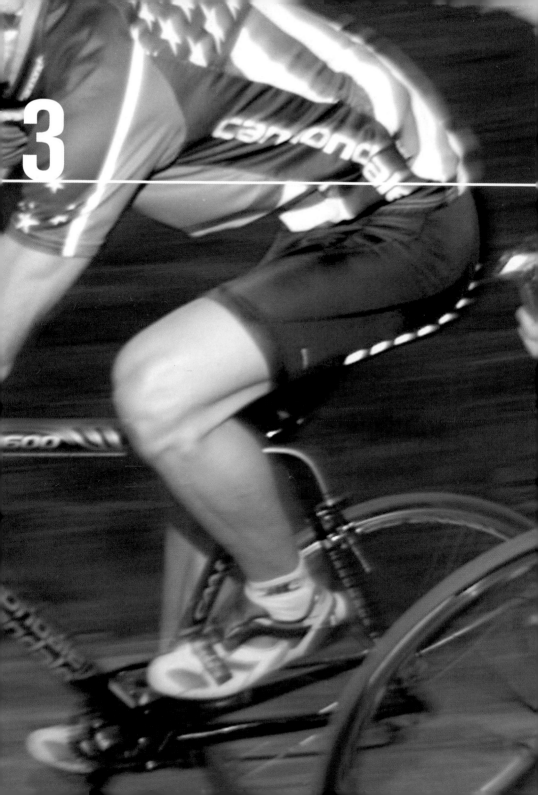

3

how to...

In this final section, you will find hints and tips covering a variety of topics, from weight loss to changing a punctured tire. There are specially designed time-saving training sessions for those really busy days, and even a short glossary to help you understand cycling jargon a little better. And if you learn one thing, make it this: enjoying your riding on your terms is success enough. Have fun.

...make the most of your time

The daily pressures of work and family life can make it difficult to find the time to enjoy life's simple pleasures, such as riding your bike. It's a hard fact to accept. If you want to fit in a ride, you may have to make some sacrifices, whether it's an extra hour in bed or the TV soap you're addicted to. Here are six suggestions to help you fit it all in.

1 Get up earlier
Morning training is a great way to start the day. It'll wake you up and energize you for the rest of the day (remember to eat before and after your ride, though). In summer, morning sessions allow you to avoid the heat of the day. In winter, they can be done in the warm comfort of your own home on your indoor trainer (see pp. 54–55).

2 Train at lunchtime
Make a habit of going to the gym on your lunch hour. You can fit in a useful weight-training session or even a quick tempo ride (15 minutes warm-up, 20 minutes tempo, 15 minutes cool-down) in that time.

3 Commute by bike
Escape the tyranny of the car and save money by commuting to work on your bike. You can even do your training sessions during your commute if you have a clear route. If not, start your training ride early, stop at home to grab a bagel and your bag, then use the ride to work as your cool-down. Alternatively, use your ride home as the warm-up for an evening session.

4 Train in the living room
If you can't get a babysitter, but you want to train, don't worry. Set your indoor trainer up in the living room and do an endurance ride while the kids watch TV or play.

5 Focus on quality
When time is short, sacrifice your recovery sessions and make an effort to get your quality rides (speed work, tempo, and so on) completed. If it means you have to do two quality days back-to-back, do the hardest first (for example, speed work), then move to the easier session the next day, then take a day off to recover.

6 Mix it up
Another way to add quality miles to your training is to do sessions within other sessions. The easiest way to do this is to do steady, tempo intervals, speed work, or sprints within your long endurance ride, but there are a number of other possibilities (see panel).

time saving sessions

1 tempo

Do some 5–15 minute tempo efforts toward the end of your steady or endurance ride.

2 speed work

Do a pyramid session of 1, 2, 3, 4, 5, 4, 3, 2, 1 minute efforts with 2-minute recoveries. Maintain the same pace until the longest effort (5 minutes). Then, make the efforts on the way back down (to 1 minute) successively harder.

3 sprints

Do speed work intervals but add a short 15-second sprint at the end of each effort (hard but very effective). Or do your sprints toward the end of your endurance or steady ride.

4 strength

Ride all the climbs on your endurance route in a flat-ground gear (for example, 52:19) at 50 to 70 rpm. Recover on the downhills and flat by spinning a small gear.

5 all-in-one

Here's one very tough but very effective all-in-one hard training session. Do not attempt it unless you have reached the level four training plans, and don't do it more than once every two weeks:

Ride 8 minutes steady. Follow that immediately with 6 minutes tempo. Then, go straight into 4 minutes hard speed work. Finish up with 2 minutes very hard, building to a sprint in the final 10 seconds, if you have the energy!

...manage your weight

It's a well-documented and acknowledged fact that the population of the western world is getting fatter. Junk food, sedentary jobs, driving everywhere, and evenings in front of the TV are all to blame. So it's no surprise that many people consider exercise as a way to manage their weight. If you want to shed a few pounds (which, if done correctly, will also make you a more efficient cyclist), here's how to do it.

power supply

Despite all the fad diets, slimming supplements, and fat-burning tools on the market, the basic principle behind losing and managing your weight is simple—eat slightly less than you burn. Aim to eat 500 kcal less than you use during the day. That way you'll be able to lose weight and still ride well. (To work out how many calories you need per day, see pp. 26–27.)

do you need to lose weight?

The best way to see whether you need to lose weight is with a body-fat test. This can be done at your gym or by your doctor, using various tests. Here's how the different percentages are categorized.

Classification	Women (% fat)	Men (% fat)
Essential Fat	10–12 percent	2–4 percent
Athletes	14–20 percent	6–13 percent
Fitness	21–24 percent	14–17 percent
Acceptable	25–31 percent	18–25 percent
Obese	32 percent plus	25 percent plus

(from the American Council For Exercise)

weight management

Take it slowly

You may be full of zeal to revamp your diet. But don't try to do everything at once. Make one change per week (for example, substitute two pieces of fruit for your mid-afternoon chocolate bar).

Don't diet

Severely restricting your food intake will leave you with very little energy for riding. If you want to lose weight, change what you eat before you change how much. Be patient and the weight will come off.

Plan your food intake

Decide what you're going to eat every morning, then stick to the plan. Set yourself a goal each month (for example, lose three pounds and eat a salad every evening) and make a note of it in your training diary.

Ride regularly

Consistent training burns calories and builds muscle. Get into a regular routine (using the training plans in Chapter 2), combine it with a controlled daily diet, and any excess weight will slowly come off.

Eat around training

Make your biggest meal of the day the one immediately after your ride. The two hours after training are when your body is most in need of refueling.

Eat breakfast

A good breakfast is essential. It will kick-start your metabolism and stop you from heading to the candy store. Aim for 400 to 500 kcal. That's a bowl of cereal with milk, a small yogurt, and a couple of pieces of fruit.

Drink lots of water

Proper hydration is vital for proper training. However, it's also a useful weight management tool because a stomach full of liquid will feel full and this will suppress hunger pangs.

Eat frequently

Studies have shown that the most efficient way to eat is to "graze"—eating little and often. This keeps blood sugar levels stable, preventing sudden cravings for food. Aim to eat five or six small meals per day.

Know thyself

While it's more efficient to eat frequent, small meals, it's also good to know how much you eat. Don't confuse eating more frequently with simply eating more. If your grazing tends to include chocolate bars and chips, you might be better off eating three healthy meals and cutting out all snacks.

Dine early

Try to eat supper several hours before you go to bed, ideally no later than 8.30pm. The body has a tendency to store more unused food as fat during the night.

and finally...

There is more to cycling than can be covered in this book, so consider asking more experienced riders for advice, or even get some coaching. But, in the meantime, below are the two most basic skills every rider must have.

...how to change a tire

1 Insert two tire levers into the rim of your wheel about 4 in (10 cm) apart and hook them under the bead of the tire.

2 Press down on the levers (toward the center of the wheel) until the tire bead pops out of the rim.

3 Run one lever around the rim to release the rest of that side of the tire.

4 Pull out the damaged inner tube and replace it with a spare (always carry a spare inner when riding).

5 Partially inflate the new tube and push it inside the tire (start at the valve, inserting it into the wheel first, then rolling the inner up into the tire).

6 Push the bead of the tire back into the rim, taking care not to pinch any of the inner. Pump up the tire.

...how to look like a pro

1 You may never be able to ride alongside Lance Armstrong up the Alp d'Huez in the Tour de France, but that doesn't mean you can't try to emulate his style and skill. Think about how you look. Is your bike well cared for? After all, you did spend a lot of money on it.

2 Also, have you shaved your legs? For ladies, this is usually a normal thing to do, so it is no problem, but for guys, it may seem a little strange. There's no law against being a hairy legged cyclist, but smooth legs move more easily through the air than hairy ones. If you do decide to go smooth, it's worth swallowing your pride and asking a woman for advice; otherwise you're going to end up cutting yourself.

3 The final aspect of emulating the pros is developing your bike control skills. Take your bike to a grassy area after a ride and practice balancing on the pedals while not moving (known as track stands), riding with no hands (eventually you'll be able to ride along like this while you put on a waterproof!), and, most importantly, falling off safely (go limp and tuck your head in as you would for a forward roll).

glossary

700C The most common road-bike wheel size, which surprisingly, almost never measures 27.6 in (700 mm) in diameter.

AERO BARS Handle bars that allow riders to rest on their forearms in a more aerodynamic position.

BAR-END SHIFTER A gear lever that mounts on the end of the handlebar. Often used on aero bars.

BEADS The two edges of a clincher-type tire. They tuck into the wheel rim to hold the tire on.

BIDON A plastic water bottle. The standard racing size carries about 1 pint (500 ml).

BONK A condition that occurs when the body's glycogen reserves are used up.

BOTTOM BRACKET The bearings and spindle to which the cranks are attached.

BREAKAWAY A group of riders who increase their pace, breaking away from the pack, so that the rest of the field cannot keep up.

BREVET A long-distance touring ride with a set time limit.

CADENCE The rate at which you turn the pedals, often measured in revolutions per minute (rpm).

CALIPER The pincer-like brake unit on the wheel. Try to get the dual, not single, pivot type.

CHAIN STAYS Tubes connecting the bottom bracket to the rear wheel.

CLEAT The plastic or metal plate attached to the underside of a cycling shoe that clips into the pedal.

CLINCHER A tire that requires a separate inner tube.

CLIPLESS PEDAL A pedal designed to lock onto a protruding cleat on the bottom of a cycling shoe.

CLUSTER A matched set of sprockets.

COL French for mountain pass. Used to describe a long mountain climb by European cyclists.

DERAILLEUR The mechanical parts that move the chain between chain rings and sprockets, respectively, to change gear. Also called mechs.

DROPOUTS Slots on the frame into which the wheel axle is clamped.

FALSE FLAT A very slight gradient that looks deceptively flat.

FIXED GEAR A bicycle on which you can't freewheel. It usually has only one gear.

FLOAT The amount of lateral movement the shoe has in a clipless pedal.

FREEWHEEL The ratchet mechanism that allows the rear wheel to turn without also turning the pedals.

GROUP, GRUPPO, GROUPSET The moving components added to a frame, such as derailleurs, chain, and brakes.

HUB The central unit of a wheel. Houses the wheel bearings and the spindle.

PACE LINE (or chain gang) A group of riders taking turns on the front.

PELOTON The pack of riders who make up the main group in a race.

RIM The outer part of a wheel that holds the tire.

SEAT POST The tube onto which the saddle is attached.

SEAT STAYS The frame tubes connecting the seat tube to the rear wheel.

STAGE RACE A race over several days. The winner is the rider with the lowest total time.

TOURING Long-distance, non-competitive leisure riding.

TRUING Making a wheel round and run straight by adjusting the tension of the spokes.

TUBULAR (or tub) A one-piece inner-tube/tire, light and often high pressure. Most often used in professional racing.

VELODROME A stadium for track races. Usually oval with heavily banked turns.

index

acknowledgments

Special thanks to Mike Cotty at Cannondale (www.cannondale.com) and Bike and Run (www.bikeand run.co.uk); many thanks also to Sweatshop for kindly providing clothing and equipment.

Thanks also to the model Leonidas Mezilis.

Additional photography: Mike Good

Every effort has been made to credit everybody who appears in this book, and we apologize in advance for any unintentional omissions. We would be pleased to insert the appropriate acknowledgment in any subsequent edition of this publication.